BREAST CANCER COOKBOOK

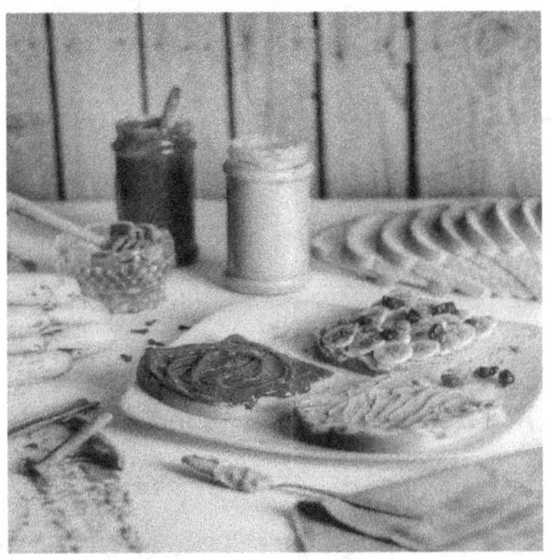

"Savoring Wellness: A Culinary Guide for Nourishing Body and Spirit during the Breast Cancer Journey With Over 30 Delicious Recipe"

EMMA LYNCH

TABLE OF CONTENTS

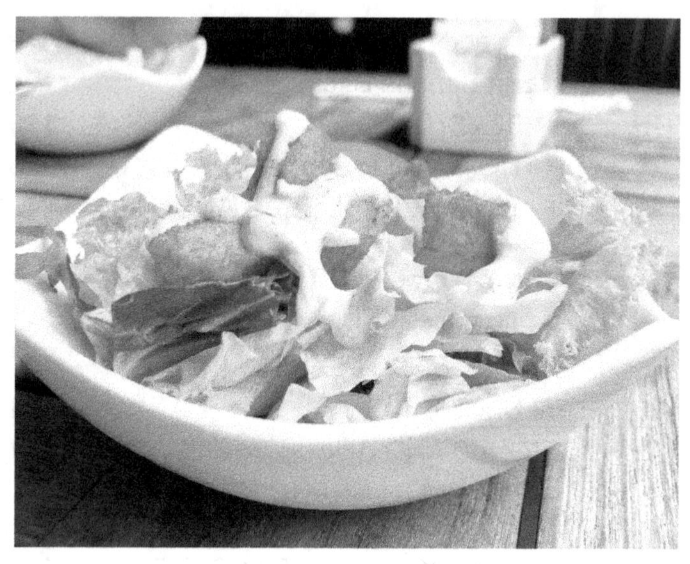

INTRODUCTION

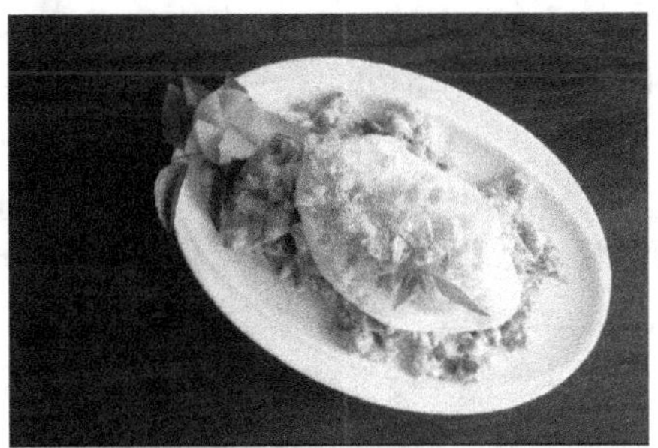

"Welcome to 'Breast cancer Cookbook: A Culinary Journey through Breast Cancer,' a heartfelt and empowering culinary guide designed to support women on their path to wellness. This cookbook is more than a collection of recipes; it's a compassionate companion tailored to the specific needs of those navigating the challenges of breast cancer.

In these pages, you will discover a symphony of flavors, carefully curated to not only tantalize your taste buds but also to address the nutritional demands that arise during this transformative journey. We understand that each woman's experience with breast cancer is unique, and so is her relationship with food. 'Breast cancer cookbook' aims to celebrate this diversity, offering a variety of recipes that cater to different dietary preferences, sensitivities, and stages of treatment.

Beyond the kitchen, this cookbook aspires to be a source of solace and inspiration. We delve into the significance of nutrition during treatment, providing insights into key nutrients, dietary guidelines, and practical tips for meal planning. It's a holistic approach, acknowledging the integral role that food plays in nurturing both the body and the spirit.

Join us on this culinary expedition, where every dish is crafted with care, understanding, and the belief that good nutrition is a vital ally in the journey to recovery. 'Breast cancer cookbook' is not just about sustenance; it's about embracing life with flavors that resonate with hope, resilience, and the determination to thrive beyond breast cancer."

OVERVIEW OF BREAST CANCER

One type of cancer that starts in the breast cells is called breast cancer. Although it can happen to men as well as women, it affects women much more frequently. The disease usually originates in the milk-producing glands (lobules) or the ducts that transport milk from the glands to the nipple. Over time, cancerous cells can invade nearby tissues and potentially spread to other parts of the body through the lymphatic system.

Risk factors for breast cancer include gender, age, family history, certain gene mutations (such as BRCA1 and BRCA2), hormonal factors, and exposure to estrogen. While some risk factors are beyond control, lifestyle factors such as maintaining a healthy weight, regular exercise, limiting alcohol consumption, and avoiding hormone replacement therapy can contribute to risk reduction.

Symptoms of breast cancer may include a lump in the breast or underarm, changes in breast size or shape, unexplained pain, skin changes on the breast, or nipple discharge other than breast milk. Early detection through regular screenings, such as mammograms and self-exams, is crucial for successful treatment.

Treatment approaches vary based on the type and stage of breast cancer but often involve a combination of surgery, radiation, chemotherapy, hormone therapy, and targeted therapy. Advances in research and medical interventions have significantly improved the prognosis for many individuals diagnosed with breast cancer, emphasizing the importance of comprehensive care and ongoing support. Regular check-ups and a multidisciplinary approach involving healthcare professionals like oncologists, surgeons, and support services contribute to a holistic and personalized approach to breast cancer management.

IMPORTANCE OF NUTRITION DURING BREAST CANCER

Nutrition plays a pivotal role in the comprehensive care and well-being of individuals facing breast cancer. The importance of proper nutrition during this journey cannot be overstated, as it contributes significantly to both physical and emotional aspects of health.

1. **Supporting Treatment Effectiveness:** A well-balanced diet can enhance the effectiveness of various cancer treatments, including surgery, chemotherapy, and radiation therapy. Proper nutrition helps the body withstand the rigors of treatment, potentially reducing complications and supporting a more robust response to therapy.

2. **Boosting Immune Function:** Nutrient-rich foods bolster the immune system, crucial for individuals undergoing cancer treatment. A strong immune system is essential for the body's ability to defend against infections and cope with the side effects of treatments.

3. **Maintaining Energy Levels:** Cancer treatments can often lead to fatigue. Adequate nutrition, including a balance of carbohydrates, proteins, and healthy fats, provides the energy necessary to combat fatigue and maintain daily activities.

4. **Managing Side Effects:** Certain foods and dietary strategies can help manage common side effects of cancer treatments, such as nausea, taste changes, and appetite loss. Tailoring the diet to individual preferences and sensitivities can improve the overall eating experience.

5. **Supporting Emotional Well-being:** The act of preparing and enjoying nourishing meals can have positive effects on emotional well-being. Food can be a source of comfort, and thoughtful, well-prepared dishes contribute to a sense of normalcy and pleasure during a challenging time.

6. **Optimizing Healing and Recovery:** Nutrition is integral to the healing process. It supports tissue repair, reduces the risk of infections, and aids in the recovery of the body after surgery or other invasive treatments.

In essence, the importance of nutrition during breast cancer extends beyond the physical; it becomes a fundamental element in the overall strategy for maintaining health, resilience, and a sense of control amid the challenges of diagnosis and treatment.

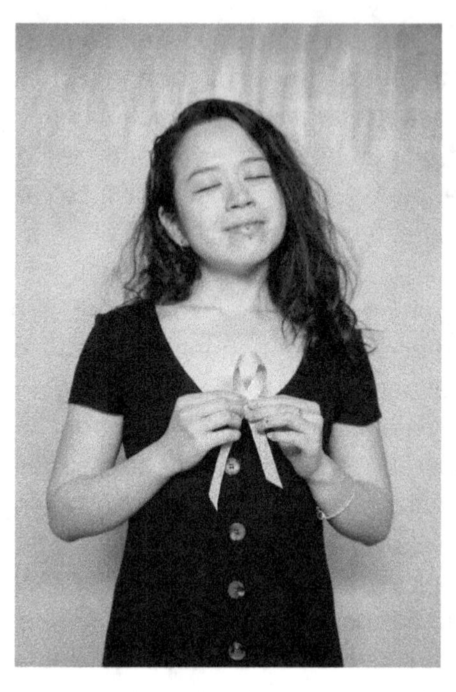

CHAPTER ONE

UNDERSTANDING NUTRITIONAL NEEDS

Understanding the nutritional needs of individuals facing breast cancer is a key aspect of promoting overall health and well-being during their journey. Tailoring dietary choices to address specific requirements can have a profound impact on treatment outcomes and quality of life.

1. **Protein for Healing and Strength:** Adequate protein intake is crucial for healing tissues and maintaining muscle strength, especially during and after treatments. Lean sources of protein, such as poultry, fish, beans, and tofu, contribute to the body's repair mechanisms.

2. **Balancing Macronutrients:** Maintaining a well-balanced ratio of macronutrients—carbohydrates, proteins, and fats—supports energy levels and overall health. Choosing complex carbohydrates, lean proteins, and healthy fats ensures a steady and sustained release of energy.

3. **Micronutrients for Immune Support:** Vitamins and minerals, such as vitamin C, vitamin D, and zinc, play essential roles in supporting the immune

system. A diet rich in fruits, vegetables, whole grains, and nuts provides a spectrum of micronutrients vital for immune function.

4. **Hydration for Vitality:** Staying well-hydrated is paramount, especially during cancer treatment. Proper hydration supports the body's ability to cope with side effects, aids in digestion, and helps maintain overall vitality.

5. **Managing Weight and Body Composition:** Balancing calorie intake with energy expenditure is crucial for managing weight, which can be challenging during breast cancer treatment. Nutrient-dense foods help meet nutritional needs without excessive caloric intake.

6. **Dietary Guidelines and Restrictions:** Understanding any dietary guidelines or restrictions recommended by healthcare professionals is essential. Some treatments may come with specific dietary considerations, and being aware of these guidelines ensures optimal support for the treatment plan.

7. **Personalized Approaches:** Recognizing the individuality of nutritional needs is key. Preferences, tolerances, and cultural considerations all play a role in creating a personalized and sustainable dietary plan.

In essence, comprehending the nutritional needs during breast cancer involves a holistic approach, considering the specific challenges of treatment, individual preferences, and the goal of promoting resilience and overall health. Working collaboratively with healthcare professionals and registered dietitians ensures a tailored and effective nutritional strategy for each individual's unique journey.

KEY NUTRIENTS FOR BREAST CANCER PATIENT

Breast cancer patients benefit from a diet rich in key nutrients that support overall health, enhance treatment effectiveness, and aid in recovery. Here are some essential nutrients to focus on:

1. **Protein:** Crucial for tissue repair and maintaining muscle mass. Sources include lean meats, poultry, fish, eggs, dairy, beans, and tofu.

2. **Omega-3 Fatty Acids:** Found in fatty fish (such as salmon and mackerel), flaxseeds, chia seeds, and walnuts, these fats have anti-inflammatory properties and support heart health.

3. **Antioxidants (Vitamins C and E, Selenium):** Protect cells from damage caused by free radicals.

Citrus fruits, berries, nuts, seeds, and whole grains are excellent sources.

4. **Calcium and Vitamin D:** Important for bone health, especially if treatments may impact bone density. Dairy products, leafy greens, fortified plant-based milk, and exposure to sunlight contribute to these nutrients.

5. **Fiber:** Aids in digestion and supports a healthy gut. Fruits, vegetables, whole grains, and legumes are all good sources.

6. **Iron:** Helps prevent anemia and supports energy levels. Include lean meats, poultry, fish, fortified cereals, and dark leafy greens in the diet.

7. **Zinc:** Supports the immune system and aids in wound healing. Foods like lean meats, dairy, nuts, and legumes provide zinc.

8. **Folate:** Important for cell division and DNA synthesis. Leafy greens, citrus fruits, avocados, and legumes are good sources.

9. **Hydration:** Staying well-hydrated is vital, especially during treatments. Water, herbal teas, and hydrating foods like fruits and vegetables contribute to fluid intake.

10. **Probiotics:** Found in fermented foods like yogurt, kefir, and sauerkraut, these support gut

health and may help manage treatment-related digestive issues.

Individual nutritional needs can vary, and it's essential to work with healthcare professionals, including a registered dietitian, to tailor dietary recommendations to the specific circumstances and preferences of each breast cancer patient. A balanced and nutrient-dense diet contributes to overall well-being and aids in maintaining strength and vitality throughout the treatment process.

DIETARY GUIDELINES AND RESTRICTIONS

Breast cancer patients may encounter specific dietary guidelines and restrictions during their treatment journey. While individual recommendations may vary based on factors such as treatment type, overall health, and personal preferences, some general guidelines and considerations include:

1. **Maintain a Balanced Diet:** Strive for a well-balanced diet that includes a variety of fruits, vegetables, whole grains, lean proteins, and healthy fats. This provides essential nutrients needed for overall health and recovery.

2. **Watch Caloric Intake:** Some cancer treatments may lead to changes in appetite or

metabolism. Monitoring caloric intake helps manage weight and energy levels. Opt for nutrient-dense foods to ensure adequate nutrition.

3. **Hydration is Key:** Stay well-hydrated, especially if experiencing treatment-related side effects. Adequate hydration supports overall health and can help manage certain side effects like nausea and fatigue.

4. **Limit Processed and Red Meats:** In some cases, healthcare providers may recommend limiting the intake of processed and red meats. Opt for lean protein sources like poultry, fish, beans, and tofu.

5. **Be Mindful of Dairy Products:** If lactose intolerance or digestive issues arise during treatment, consider lactose-free or plant-based alternatives for dairy products to ensure adequate calcium intake.

6. **Manage Nausea and Taste Changes:** Experiment with small, frequent meals and bland or cool foods to manage nausea. Adjusting cooking methods and exploring different flavors can help address taste changes.

7. **Consider Nutritional Supplements:** In cases where it's challenging to meet nutritional needs through food alone, healthcare providers may

recommend supplements. This could include vitamins, minerals, or other specific nutrients.

8. **Consult with a Dietitian:** Collaborate with a registered dietitian specializing in oncology to create a personalized nutrition plan. They can offer tailored advice, address dietary concerns, and ensure nutritional goals align with the treatment plan.

9. **Avoid Alcohol:** Limit or avoid alcohol consumption, as it can interact with certain medications and may increase the risk of complications during treatment.

10. **Stay Cautious with Herbal Supplements:** Inform healthcare providers about any herbal supplements, as they may interact with medications or treatments. Some herbs can interfere with the effectiveness of cancer therapies.

It's crucial for breast cancer patients to communicate openly with their healthcare team and seek guidance on dietary choices. Individualized recommendations based on medical history and treatment specifics contribute to a supportive and effective nutritional approach during the breast cancer journey.

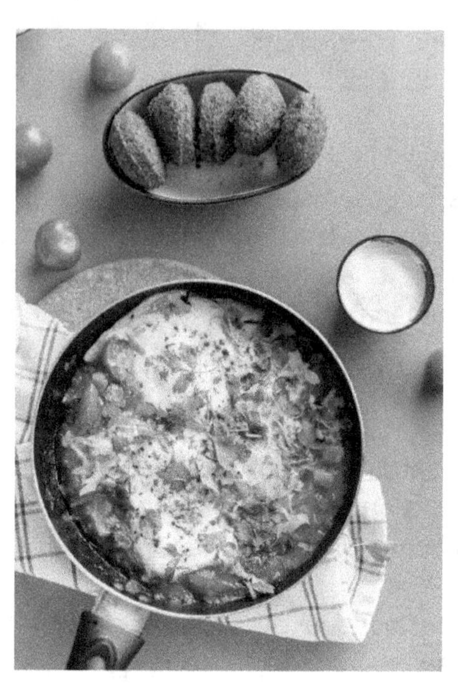

CHAPTER TWO

BREAKFAST BOOSTERS

Certainly! Here are 10 breakfast booster recipes with detailed instructions:

Berry Power Smoothie

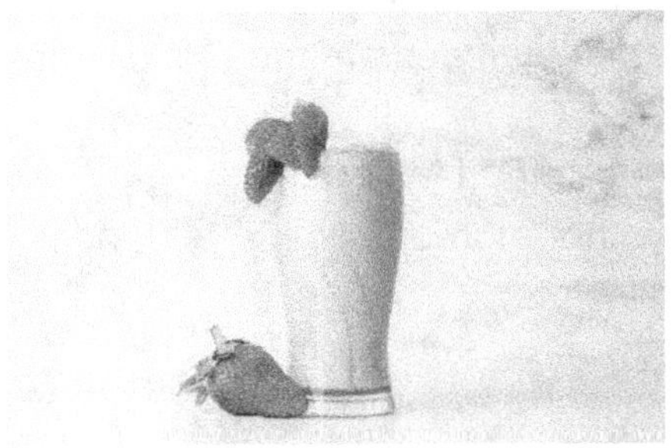

 Certainly! Here's a simple recipe for a Berry Power Smoothie:

Ingredients:
- One cup of mixed berries, including raspberries, blueberries, and strawberries
- 1 banana
- 1/2 cup Greek yogurt
- 1 tablespoon chia seeds
- 1 cup almond milk

Instructions:
1. **Prepare the Ingredients:**

- Wash the mixed berries thoroughly.
- Peel and slice the banana.

2. **Blend the Berries and Banana:**
   - In a blender, combine the mixed berries and sliced banana.

3. **Add Greek Yogurt:**
   - Spoon in the Greek yogurt into the blender.

4. **Incorporate Chia Seeds:**
   - Place the chia seeds in the blender and blend.

5. **Pour in Almond Milk:**
   - To the other ingredients in the blender, add the almond milk.

6. **Blend Until Smooth:**
   - Secure the blender lid and blend the ingredients until smooth and well combined.

7. **Check Consistency:**
   - If the smoothie is too thick, you can add more almond milk and blend again until you reach your desired consistency.

8. **Serve and Enjoy:**
   - Pour the Berry Power Smoothie into a glass.
   - Optionally, garnish with a few whole berries on top.

9. **Customize (Optional):**

   - Feel free to customize your smoothie by adding
a handful of ice cubes for a colder texture or a
drizzle of honey for added sweetness.

10. **Enjoy the Nutrient Boost:**
   - Sip and savor your Berry Power Smoothie,
packed with antioxidants, vitamins, and a delightful
burst of berry goodness.

This smoothie not only provides a delicious and
refreshing start to your day but also offers a
nutritional boost, making it a great choice for
individuals on the breast cancer journey.

Quinoa Breakfast Bowl

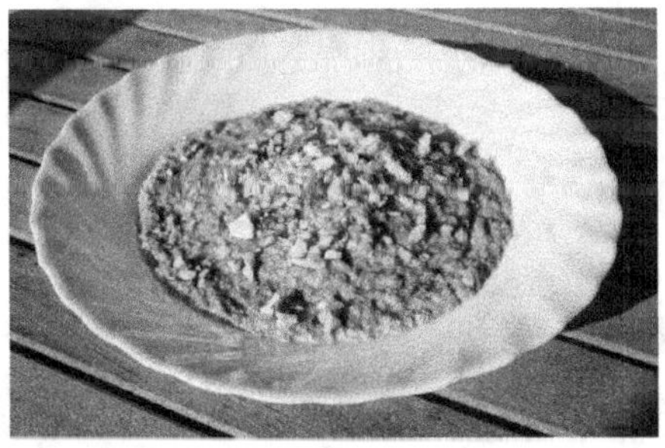

Certainly! Here's a nutritious and tasty recipe for a
Quinoa Breakfast Bowl:

Ingredients:
- 1/2 cup cooked quinoa
- 1/4 cup sliced almonds

- 1/2 cup fresh mango chunks
- 1 tablespoon honey
- 1/2 teaspoon cinnamon

Instructions:

1. **Prepare the Quinoa:**
   - Cook quinoa according to package instructions. When cooked, fluff with a fork.

2. **Toast the Almonds:**
   - In a dry skillet over medium heat, toast the sliced almonds until they become golden brown and fragrant. Be cautious not to burn them, as this can happen quickly.

3. **Assemble the Bowl:**
   - In a bowl, combine the cooked quinoa and toasted almonds.

4. **Add Fresh Mango Chunks:**
   - Gently fold in the fresh mango chunks. The sweetness of mango complements the nutty flavor of quinoa.

5. **Drizzle with Honey:**
   - Drizzle honey over the quinoa and mango mixture. Adjust the amount to suit your personal sweetness level.

6. **Sprinkle with Cinnamon:**

  - Sprinkle cinnamon over the bowl for a warm and aromatic flavor.

7. **Mix Well:**
  - Toss all the ingredients together until well combined.

8. **Serve:**
  - Spoon the quinoa breakfast bowl into your serving dish.

9. **Customize (Optional):**
  - Feel free to customize your bowl by adding a dollop of Greek yogurt, a sprinkle of additional nuts or seeds, or a few extra slices of fresh fruit.

10. **Enjoy the Nutrient-Rich Breakfast:**
  - Delight in your Quinoa Breakfast Bowl, a nutritious blend of whole grains, healthy fats, and natural sweetness. It's a satisfying and energy-boosting way to start your day.

This breakfast bowl not only provides a hearty and filling meal but also offers a variety of nutrients, making it an excellent choice for individuals seeking a nourishing breakfast during the breast cancer journey.

Avocado and Egg Toast

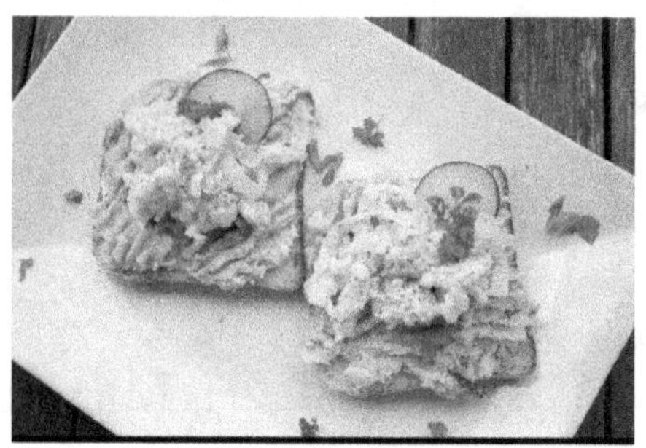

Certainly! Here's a simple and nutritious recipe for Avocado and Egg Toast:

Ingredients:
- 1 slice whole-grain bread
- 1/2 ripe avocado, mashed
- 1 poached egg
- Salt and pepper to taste

Instructions:

1. **Toast the Bread:**
   - Toast the whole-grain bread to your preferred level of crispiness.

2. **Prepare the Avocado:**
   - While the bread is toasting, cut the avocado in half, remove the pit, and scoop out the flesh into a bowl.

3. **Mash the Avocado:**

- Mash the avocado with a fork until you achieve a smooth consistency. Season to taste with a pinch of salt and pepper.

4. **Poach the Egg:**
   - Poach an egg to your liking. You can poach it using your preferred method - on the stovetop or using an egg poacher.

5. **Assemble the Toast:**
   - Evenly cover the toasted bread with the mashed avocado.

6. **Add the Poached Egg:**
   - On top of the mashed avocado, carefully add the poached egg.

7. **Season to Taste:**
   - Sprinkle a bit of salt and pepper over the poached egg to enhance the flavors.

8. **Optional Garnish (Optional):**
   - Optionally, garnish with a sprinkle of red pepper flakes, chives, or a dash of hot sauce for added flavor.

9. **Serve:**
   - Place the Avocado and Egg Toast on a plate or a serving board.

10. **Enjoy Your Nutrient-Packed Breakfast:**

- Relish your Avocado and Egg Toast, a wholesome combination of fiber, healthy fats, and protein. It's a satisfying and delicious breakfast that provides a good balance of nutrients.

This breakfast option not only offers a burst of flavors but also provides essential nutrients, making it an excellent choice for individuals seeking a nourishing and tasty meal during the breast cancer journey.

Greek Yogurt Parfait

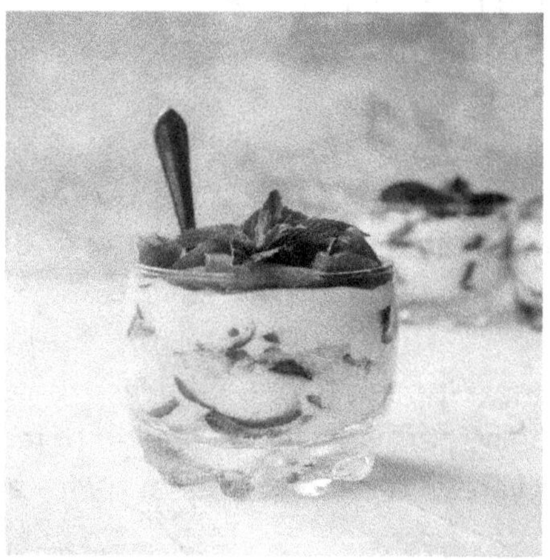

Absolutely! Here's a delightful and nutritious recipe for a Greek Yogurt Parfait:

Ingredients:
- 1 cup Greek yogurt
- 1/2 cup granola

- Half a cup of mixed berries, including raspberries, blueberries, and strawberries
- Drizzle of honey

Instructions:

1. **Choose Your Yogurt:**
   - Select your favorite flavor of Greek yogurt. Opt for plain or a lightly sweetened variety to control sugar intake.

2. **Prepare the Berries:**
   - Wash and slice strawberries, and ensure blueberries and raspberries are clean and ready to use.

3. **Layer the Yogurt:**
   - In a glass or a bowl, start by spooning a layer of Greek yogurt at the bottom.

4. **Add a Layer of Granola:**
   - Drizzle granola on top of the yogurt. Choose your favorite granola variety for added texture and crunch.

5. **Introduce the Mixed Berries:**
   - Spread some mixed berries over the granola. Spread them evenly to ensure each bite is filled with fruity goodness.

6. **Repeat Layers:**

- Until you reach the top of the glass or bowl, keep layering. The order is flexible, so feel free to customize based on your preference.

7. **Drizzle with Honey:**
   - Drizzle a bit of honey over the top for a touch of sweetness. To suit your taste, adjust the quantity.

8. **Optional Additions (Optional):**
   - Consider adding a sprinkle of nuts, seeds, or coconut flakes for extra flavor and nutrition.

9. **Serve Immediately:**
   - This Greek Yogurt Parfait is best enjoyed immediately to maintain the crispness of the granola.

10. **Enjoy Your Wholesome Parfait:**
    - Delight in the layers of creamy yogurt, crunchy granola, and vibrant berries. The Greek Yogurt Parfait offers a combination of protein, fiber, and antioxidants for a nourishing start to your day.

This parfait not only provides a satisfying breakfast but also offers a beautiful balance of textures and flavors, making it an excellent choice for individuals looking for a wholesome and tasty option during the breast cancer journey.

Spinach and Feta Omelette

Certainly! Here's a simple and delicious recipe for a Spinach and Feta Omelette:

Spinach and Feta Omelette

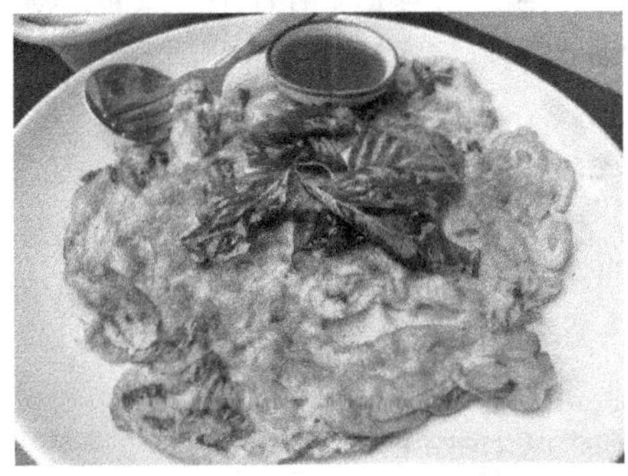

Ingredients:
- 2 eggs, beaten
- Handful of fresh spinach leaves
- 2 tablespoons crumbled feta cheese
- Salt and pepper to taste

Instructions:

1. **Prepare the Spinach:**
   - Thoroughly wash the fresh spinach leaves and wipe dry.

2. **Sauté the Spinach:**
   - In a non-stick skillet over medium heat, sauté the fresh spinach until wilted. It should just require a few minutes to complete.

3. **Beat the Eggs:**
   - In a bowl, beat the eggs until well combined. Season with a pinch of salt and pepper.

4. **Add Eggs to the Skillet:**
   - Pour the beaten eggs into the skillet with the sautéed spinach.

5. **Swirl and Cook:**
   - Gently swirl the skillet to spread the eggs evenly. Allow the eggs to cook for about a minute, or until the edges begin to firm.

6. **Add Feta Cheese:**
   - Sprinkle the crumbled feta cheese evenly over one half of the omelette.

7. **Fold the Omelette:**
   - Once the edges of the omelette are set but the center is still slightly runny, carefully fold the omelette in half, covering the side with the feta cheese.

8. **Finish Cooking:**
   - Allow the omelette to cook for an additional minute or until the center is fully set and the feta cheese is melted.

9. **Slide Onto a Plate:**
   - Slide the Spinach and Feta Omelette onto a plate, folding it onto itself.

10. **Serve Immediately:**
    - Enjoy your Spinach and Feta Omelette while it's warm. You can garnish with additional feta, herbs, or a sprinkle of black pepper if desired.

This omelette not only offers a tasty combination of spinach and feta but also provides a good dose of protein and nutrients, making it a wholesome choice for a nutritious breakfast during the breast cancer journey.

Chia Seed Pudding

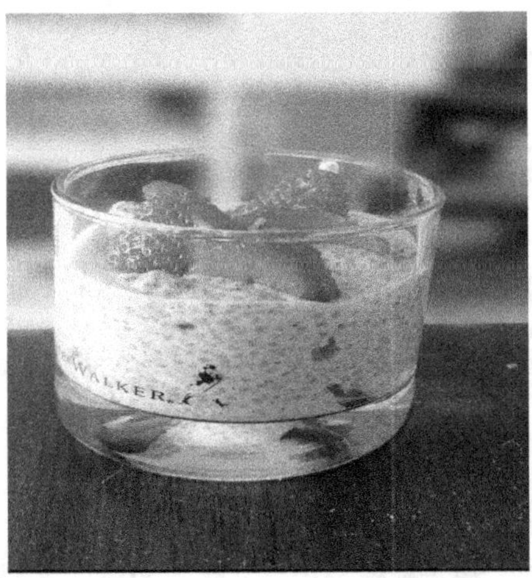

Certainly! Here's a simple recipe for Chia Seed Pudding:

Ingredients:
- 3 tablespoons chia seeds
- One cup almond milk, or any other type of milk you prefer
- 1/2 teaspoon vanilla extract
- Fresh fruit for topping (e.g., berries, sliced kiwi)

Instructions:

1. **Mix Chia Seeds and Milk:**
   - In a bowl or jar, combine the chia seeds and almond milk. Make sure the chia seeds are dispersed evenly by giving it a good stir.

2. **Add Vanilla Extract:**
   - Pour in the vanilla extract and mix it into the chia seed and milk mixture.

3. **Stir Again:**
   - Stir the ingredients thoroughly to prevent clumping. Make sure the chia seeds are well incorporated into the liquid.

4. **Refrigerate:**
   - Cover the bowl or jar and place it in the refrigerator. Let it sit for at least 2-3 hours or, ideally, overnight. This enables the liquid to be

absorbed by the chia seeds, giving the mixture a pudding-like consistency.

5. **Check and Stir:**
   - After the initial refrigeration period, check the pudding. Stir it to break up any clumps and ensure an even texture.

6. **Top with Fresh Fruit:**
   - When ready to serve, top the chia seed pudding with your favorite fresh fruits. Berries, sliced kiwi, and mango are excellent choices.

7. **Optional Additions (Optional):**
   - Customize your chia seed pudding by adding a drizzle of honey, a sprinkle of nuts, or a dash of cinnamon for added flavor.

8. **Serve Chilled:**
   - Scoop the Chia Seed Pudding into serving bowls or glasses. It's best enjoyed cold.

9. **Enjoy the Nutrient-Rich Pudding:**
   - Indulge in this nutritious and satisfying Chia Seed Pudding, packed with omega-3 fatty acids, fiber, and a delightful blend of textures.

This pudding not only serves as a delicious breakfast or snack option but also provides a good source of energy and essential nutrients during the breast cancer journey.

Peanut Butter Banana Toast

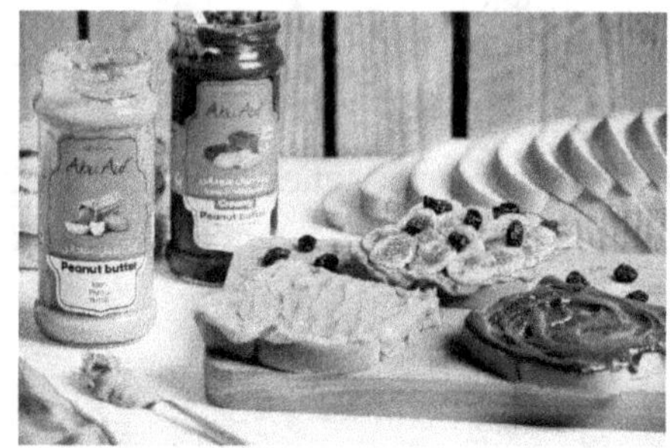

  Certainly! Here's a quick and tasty recipe for Peanut Butter Banana Toast:

Ingredients:
- 1 slice whole-grain bread
- 1 tablespoon peanut butter
- 1 banana, sliced
- Drizzle of honey (optional)

Instructions:

1. **Toast the Bread:**
   - Toast the slice of whole-grain bread to your desired level of crispiness.

2. **Spread Peanut Butter:**
   - While the bread is still warm, spread the peanut butter evenly over the entire surface.

3. **Slice the Banana:**
   - Peel the banana and slice it into thin rounds.

4. **Arrange Banana Slices:**
   - Arrange the banana slices on top of the peanut butter-covered toast.

5. **Optional Drizzle of Honey:**
   - If you desire a touch of sweetness, drizzle a bit of honey over the banana slices. Adapt the quantity to your personal taste.

6. **Serve Immediately:**
   - Serve the Peanut Butter Banana Toast while it's warm.

7. **Optional Garnish (Optional):**
   - Optionally, garnish with a sprinkle of cinnamon or a few crushed nuts for added flavor and texture.

8. **Enjoy Your Nutrient-Packed Toast:**
   - Savor this delicious and satisfying Peanut Butter Banana Toast, combining the creaminess of peanut butter with the natural sweetness of bananas.

This quick and easy recipe provides a delightful combination of protein, healthy fats, and natural sugars, making it a wholesome choice for a tasty breakfast or snack during the breast cancer journey.

Blueberry Almond Pancakes

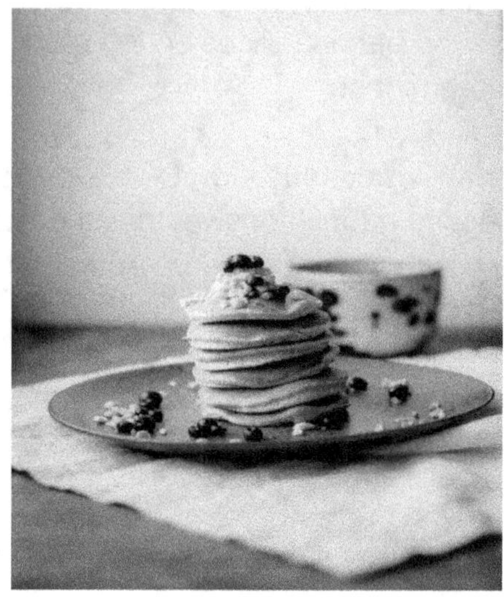

Certainly! Here's a delightful recipe for Blueberry Almond Pancakes:

Ingredients:
- 1 cup pancake mix (whole grain if preferred)
- 1/2 cup almond milk
- 1/2 cup fresh blueberries
- Sliced almonds for garnish

Instructions:

1. **Prepare Pancake Batter:**
   - In a mixing bowl, combine the pancake mix and almond milk. Until the batter is smooth, stir.

2. **Fold in Blueberries:**

- Stir in the fresh blueberries gently into the pancake mixture. Ensure even distribution.

3. **Heat the Griddle or Pan:**
   - Preheat a griddle or nonstick skillet on medium heat. Cooking spray or a tiny amount of oil should be used to lightly grease the surface.

4. **Pour Batter onto Griddle:**
   - Pour ladlefuls of pancake batter onto the hot griddle, forming circles of the desired size.

5. **Cook Until Bubbles Form:**
   - Allow the pancakes to cook until you see bubbles forming on the surface. This usually takes 2-3 minutes.

6. **Flip the Pancakes:**
   - Carefully flip the pancakes using a spatula. Cook the other side until it's golden brown.

7. **Repeat:**
   - Repeat the process until you've used all the batter, making a stack of delicious blueberry pancakes.

8. **Serve:**
   - The pancakes should be put on a serving plate.

9. **Garnish with Almonds:**
   - Sprinkle sliced almonds on top of the pancakes for a delightful crunch and added flavor.

10. **Optional Toppings (Optional):**
   - Serve with additional fresh blueberries, a drizzle of maple syrup, or a dollop of Greek yogurt if desired.

11. **Enjoy Your Blueberry Almond Pancakes:**
   - Indulge in these light and fluffy Blueberry Almond Pancakes, a delightful combination of nuttiness and bursts of sweetness from the blueberries.

This pancake recipe not only makes for a delicious breakfast but also incorporates the nutritional benefits of whole grains, almonds, and antioxidant-rich blueberries, making it a wholesome choice for individuals on the breast cancer journey.

Smoked Salmon Bagel

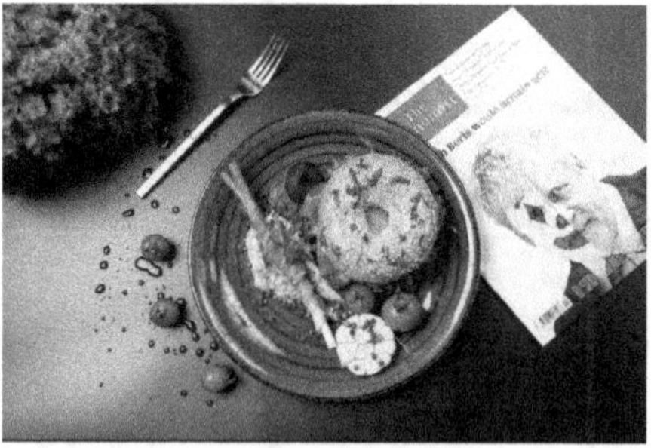

Certainly! Here's a simple and delicious recipe for Smoked Salmon Bagel:

Ingredients:
- 1 whole-grain bagel, toasted
- 2 tablespoons cream cheese
- Smoked salmon slices
- Capers and red onion slices for topping

Instructions:

1. **Toast the Bagel:**
   - Toast the whole-grain bagel until it reaches your preferred level of crispiness.

2. **Spread Cream Cheese:**
   - While the bagel is still warm, spread cream cheese evenly on both halves.

3. **Layer with Smoked Salmon:**
   - Place slices of smoked salmon generously on top of the cream cheese.

4. **Add Capers and Red Onion:**
   - Sprinkle capers and place thin slices of red onion on the smoked salmon. These ingredients add a burst of flavor and complement the richness of the salmon.

5. **Optional Garnish (Optional):**
   - Optionally, garnish with fresh dill or a squeeze of lemon juice for added freshness.

6. **Assemble and Serve:**

- Bring the two halves of the bagel together, creating a delicious and visually appealing Smoked Salmon Bagel sandwich.

7. **Enjoy Your Gourmet Bagel:**
   - Indulge in the flavors of this Smoked Salmon Bagel, a classic combination that offers a balance of creaminess, smokiness, and a touch of brininess.

This bagel recipe not only makes for a delightful breakfast or brunch option but also provides a good source of omega-3 fatty acids from the smoked salmon, making it a nutritious and flavorful choice during the breast cancer journey.

Turmeric and Ginger Smoothie Bowl

Certainly! Here's a refreshing recipe for a Turmeric and Ginger Smoothie Bowl:

Ingredients:

- 1 frozen banana
- 1/2 teaspoon turmeric powder
- 1/2 teaspoon grated ginger
- One cup coconut milk, or any other type of milk you prefer
- Toppings: Granola, sliced kiwi, coconut flakes

Instructions:

1. **Prepare the Ingredients:**
   - Peel and slice the banana before freezing it in advance.

2. **Blend the Smoothie Base:**
   - In a blender, combine the frozen banana slices, turmeric powder, grated ginger, and coconut milk.

3. **Blend Until Smooth:**
   - The ingredients should be blended until a creamy and smooth consistency is reached. Add more milk if needed.

4. **Adjust Consistency (Optional):**
   - If the smoothie is too thick, you can add a little more coconut milk and blend again until you reach your desired consistency.

5. **Pour into a Bowl:**
   - Pour the turmeric and ginger smoothie into a bowl.

6. **Top with Toppings:**
   - Sprinkle granola over the smoothie bowl for crunch. Add sliced kiwi and coconut flakes for extra flavor and texture.

7. **Optional Additions (Optional):**

- Feel free to add other toppings like chia seeds, sliced almonds, or a drizzle of honey for additional sweetness.

8. **Serve Immediately:**
   - Enjoy your Turmeric and Ginger Smoothie Bowl immediately while it's fresh and chilled.

9. **Savor the Nutrient-Packed Bowl:**
   - Delight in this vibrant and nutrient-packed smoothie bowl, rich in antioxidants and anti-inflammatory properties from turmeric and ginger.

This smoothie bowl not only provides a refreshing and flavorful start to your day but also incorporates the health benefits of turmeric and ginger, making it a nourishing choice during the breast cancer journey.

Enjoy these nourishing and flavorful breakfast options tailored to boost your morning and support your well-being during the breast cancer journey.

CHAPTER THREE

NOURISHING LUNCHES

Certainly! Here are eight nourishing lunch ideas that offer a balance of flavors and essential nutrients:

Grilled Chicken Salad Bowl

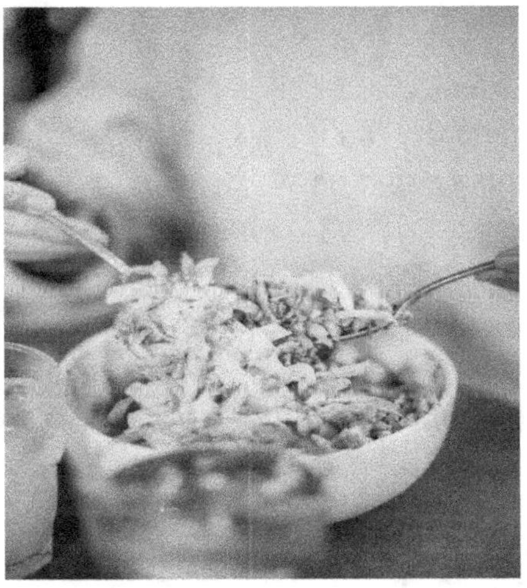

Certainly! Here's a delicious recipe for a Grilled Chicken Salad Bowl:

Ingredients:
- Grilled chicken breast slices
- Mixed greens (spinach, arugula, kale)
- Cherry tomatoes, halved

- Cucumber slices
- Avocado chunks
- Quinoa or brown rice (optional)
- Balsamic vinaigrette dressing

Instructions:

1. **Grill the Chicken:**
   - Season chicken breasts with your favorite herbs and spices. Grill until fully cooked, ensuring a nice char on the outside. Grilled chicken should be cut into tiny strips.

2. **Prepare the Greens:**
   - Wash and dry the mixed greens. After that, move to a big salad bowl.

3. **Add Fresh Vegetables:**
   - Slice cherry tomatoes in half and add them to the greens.
   - Arrange cucumber slices and avocado chunks on top.

4. **Include Whole Grains (Optional):**
   - For added substance, include a serving of cooked quinoa or brown rice. This step is optional but provides additional nutrients and fiber.

5. **Top with Grilled Chicken:**
   - Place the grilled chicken slices on top of the salad.

6. **Drizzle with Dressing:**
   - Drizzle the salad with balsamic vinaigrette dressing. Use a light hand initially, and add more according to your taste preferences.

7. **Toss Gently:**
   - Gently toss the salad to ensure all ingredients are well mixed and coated with the dressing.

8. **Serve Immediately:**
   - Divide the salad into individual bowls or plates and serve immediately.

9. **Customize (Optional):**
   - Customize your grilled chicken salad bowl by adding nuts, seeds, or crumbled feta cheese for extra flavor and texture.

10. **Enjoy Your Nourishing Salad:**
    - Indulge in this Grilled Chicken Salad Bowl, a nutrient-rich and satisfying meal that combines the goodness of lean protein, vibrant vegetables, and a flavorful dressing.

This salad bowl not only offers a burst of flavors but also provides a well-balanced combination of proteins, healthy fats, and a variety of vitamins and minerals, making it a nourishing choice during the breast cancer journey.

Vegetarian Quinoa Stir-Fry

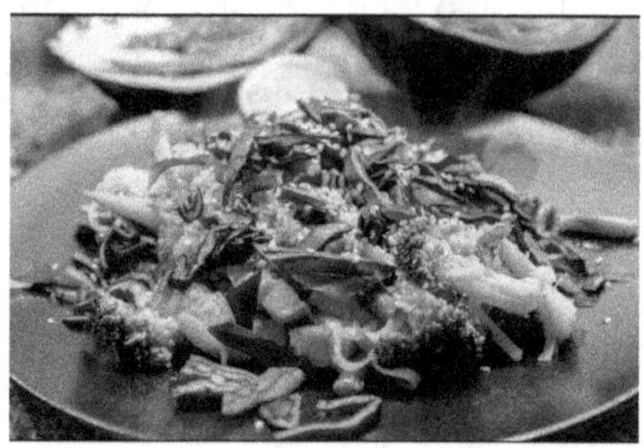

Certainly! Here's a delicious recipe for Vegetarian Quinoa Stir-Fry:

Ingredients:
- Quinoa
- Tofu or chickpeas (for protein)
- Broccoli florets
- Bell peppers (assorted colors)
- Carrot strips
- Snap peas
- Soy sauce and ginger-based stir-fry sauce

Instructions:

1. **Cook Quinoa:**
   - Rinse quinoa under cold water. Cook quinoa according to package instructions. Set aside.

2. **Prepare Tofu or Chickpeas:**

- If using tofu, press out excess water, cut it into cubes, and sauté until golden brown. If using chickpeas, drain and rinse them.

3. **Sauté Vegetables:**
   - A wok or sizable skillet should be heated to medium-high heat. Add a small amount of oil.
   - Sauté broccoli, bell peppers, carrot strips, and snap peas until they are slightly tender but still crisp.

4. **Add Tofu or Chickpeas:**
   - Add the cooked tofu or chickpeas to the vegetables in the wok.

5. **Stir-Fry Sauce:**
   - Pour a soy sauce and ginger-based stir-fry sauce over the tofu/vegetable mixture. Toss to coat evenly.

6. **Incorporate Cooked Quinoa:**
   - Add the cooked quinoa to the wok, tossing everything together until well combined.

7. **Adjust Seasoning:**
   - Taste and adjust the seasoning if needed. You can add more soy sauce or a dash of sesame oil for extra flavor.

8. **Serve Hot:**
   - Once heated through, serve the Vegetarian Quinoa Stir-Fry hot.

9. **Garnish (Optional):**
   - Garnish with chopped green onions, sesame seeds, or cilantro for an extra burst of freshness.

10. **Enjoy Your Flavorful Stir-Fry:**
   - Delight in this colorful and nutritious Vegetarian Quinoa Stir-Fry, providing a satisfying combination of protein, veggies, and whole grains.

Feel free to customize the vegetables and protein source based on your preferences. This stir-fry is not only delicious but also a great source of plant-based protein and a variety of essential nutrients.

Salmon and Sweet Potato

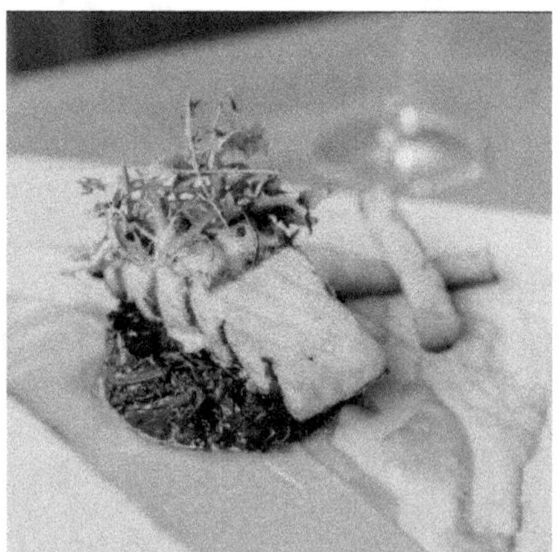

Certainly! Here's a tasty recipe for Salmon and Sweet Potato:

Ingredients:
- Salmon fillets
- Sweet potatoes, peeled and sliced into wedges
- Olive oil
- Salt and pepper to taste
- Lemon wedges for serving
- For garnish, use fresh herbs like parsley or dill.

Instructions:

1. **Preheat the Oven:**
   - Set the oven temperature to 400°F, or 200°C.

2. **Prepare Salmon:**
   - Utilizing paper towels, pat the salmon fillets dry. Add salt and pepper to both sides for seasoning.

3. **Prepare Sweet Potatoes:**
   - Add salt, pepper, and olive oil to the sweet potato wedges.

4. **Arrange on Baking Sheet:**
   - Place the seasoned salmon fillets and sweet potato wedges on a baking sheet, ensuring they are not overcrowded.

5. **Bake in the Oven:**
   - Bake in the preheated oven for about 20-25 minutes or until the salmon is cooked through and

flakes easily with a fork, and the sweet potatoes are tender.

6. **Check Doneness:**
   - Check the doneness of the sweet potatoes by inserting a fork into one. If it fits in with ease, they're prepared.

7. **Optional Broiling (Optional):**
   - If you prefer a slightly crispy texture, you can broil the salmon and sweet potatoes for an additional 2-3 minutes until the tops are golden.

8. **Serve Hot:**
   - Take the baking sheet out of the oven with care. Serve the salmon and sweet potato hot.

9. **Garnish:**
   - For extra taste, garnish with fresh herbs like parsley or dill.

10. **Serve with Lemon Wedges:**
    - Serve with lemon wedges on the side. Squeezing a bit of lemon over the salmon adds a refreshing citrus flavor.

11. **Enjoy Your Balanced Meal:**
    - Enjoy this balanced and nutritious meal of Salmon and Sweet Potato, providing a combination of healthy fats, protein, and complex carbohydrates.

This recipe is not only delicious but also rich in omega-3 fatty acids from salmon and the nutritional benefits of sweet potatoes, making it a nourishing choice during the breast cancer journey.

Mediterranean Chickpea Bowl

Certainly! Here's a flavorful recipe for a Mediterranean Chickpea Bowl:

Mediterranean Chickpea Bowl

Ingredients:
- Chickpeas (canned, drained, and rinsed)
- Quinoa or couscous, cooked
- Cherry tomatoes, halved
- Cucumber, diced
- Kalamata olives, pitted and sliced
- Feta cheese, crumbled
- Lemon juice and olive oil, or Greek dressing
- Fresh parsley, chopped (for garnish)

Instructions:

1. **Prepare Chickpeas:**
   - Drain and rinse canned chickpeas. You can sauté them in olive oil with a pinch of salt and your favorite Mediterranean spices for added flavor.

2. **Cook Quinoa or Couscous:**

   - Cook quinoa or couscous according to package
instructions. Fluff with a fork once cooked.

3. **Assemble the Base:**
   - In a bowl or plate, create a base layer with
cooked quinoa or couscous.

4. **Add Chickpeas:**
   - Spoon the sautéed chickpeas over the quinoa or
couscous.

5. **Layer with Fresh Vegetables:**
   - Add halved cherry tomatoes, diced cucumber,
and sliced Kalamata olives on top of the chickpeas.

6. **Sprinkle Feta Cheese:**
   - Over the vegetables, scatter the crumbled feta
cheese.

7. **Drizzle Dressing:**
   - Drizzle Greek dressing or a mix of olive oil and
lemon juice over the entire bowl.

8. **Toss Gently:**
   - Gently toss the ingredients to ensure even
distribution of flavors.

9. **Garnish with Fresh Parsley:**
   - Garnish the Mediterranean Chickpea Bowl with
chopped fresh parsley.

10. **Serve Immediately:**

   - Serve the bowl immediately while it's fresh and vibrant.

11. **Customize (Optional):**
   - Customize your bowl by adding additional ingredients like artichoke hearts, red onion slices, or roasted red peppers.

12. **Enjoy Your Mediterranean Delight:**
   - Delight in this Mediterranean Chickpea Bowl, a colorful and nutrient-rich dish showcasing the flavors of the Mediterranean.

This bowl not only provides a delicious combination of ingredients but also offers a variety of nutrients and antioxidants, making it a wholesome and satisfying choice during the breast cancer journey.

Caprese Wrap

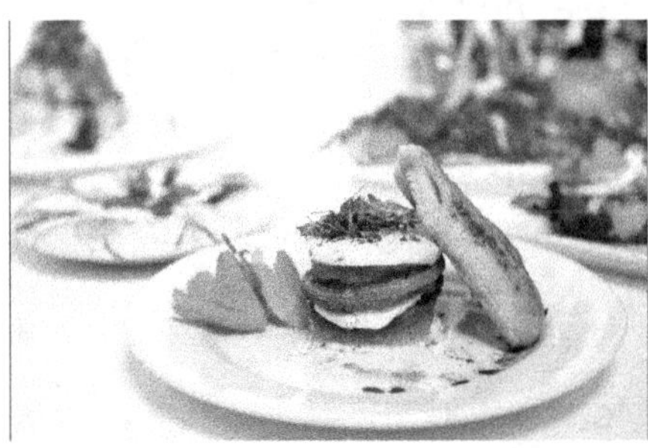

Certainly! Here's a delicious recipe for a Caprese Wrap:

Ingredients:
- Whole-grain wrap or tortilla
- Fresh tomatoes, sliced
- Fresh mozzarella cheese, sliced
- Fresh basil leaves
- Balsamic glaze or balsamic vinaigrette
- Salt and pepper to taste
- Extra-virgin olive oil (optional)

Instructions:

1. **Prepare Ingredients:**
   - Slice fresh tomatoes and fresh mozzarella cheese. Wash and dry basil leaves.

2. **Warm the Wrap:**
   - Warm the whole-grain wrap or tortilla according to package instructions or on a dry skillet for a few seconds on each side.

3. **Assemble the Wrap:**
   - Lay the warmed wrap on a flat surface.

4. **Layer Tomatoes:**
   - Arrange slices of fresh tomatoes evenly over the wrap.

5. **Add Mozzarella:**
   - Top the tomatoes with slices of fresh mozzarella cheese.

6. **Add Basil Leaves:**

- Scatter fresh basil leaves over the tomatoes and mozzarella.

7. **Season with Salt and Pepper:**
   - Sprinkle a pinch of salt and pepper over the ingredients. Adjust to taste.

8. **Drizzle Balsamic Glaze:**
   - Drizzle balsamic glaze or balsamic vinaigrette over the wrap for a burst of flavor.

9. **Optional Drizzle of Olive Oil (Optional):**
   - For added richness, you can drizzle a small amount of extra-virgin olive oil over the ingredients.

10. **Fold and Roll:**
    - Carefully fold and roll the wrap, securing the ingredients inside.

11. **Slice and Serve:**
    - Slice the Caprese Wrap in half diagonally or leave it whole. Serve immediately.

12. **Enjoy Your Fresh Caprese Wrap:**
    - Enjoy this fresh and flavorful Caprese Wrap, a delightful combination of ripe tomatoes, creamy mozzarella, and aromatic basil.

Feel free to customize your Caprese Wrap by adding extras like avocado slices, a sprinkle of pine nuts, or a handful of arugula for added texture and flavor. This recipe offers a light and nutritious option during the breast cancer journey.

Shrimp and Avocado Wrap

Certainly! Here's a tasty recipe for a Shrimp and Avocado Wrap:

Ingredients:
- Whole-grain wrap or tortilla
- Grilled or sautéed shrimp
- Ripe avocado, sliced
- Shredded lettuce
- Diced tomatoes
- Greek yogurt-based dressing or lime crema
- Salt and pepper to taste
- Fresh cilantro for garnish (optional)

Instructions:

1. **Prepare Ingredients:**
   - Grill or sauté shrimp until cooked. Slice ripe avocado, dice tomatoes, and shred lettuce.

2. **Warm the Wrap:**
   - Warm the whole-grain wrap or tortilla according to package instructions or on a dry skillet for a few seconds on each side.

3. **Assemble the Wrap:**

- Lay the warmed wrap on a flat surface.

4. **Layer Shrimp:**
   - Arrange grilled or sautéed shrimp evenly over the wrap.

5. **Add Avocado Slices:**
   - Place slices of ripe avocado on top of the shrimp.

6. **Sprinkle Lettuce and Tomatoes:**
   - Sprinkle shredded lettuce and diced tomatoes over the shrimp and avocado.

7. **Season with Salt and Pepper:**
   - Sprinkle a pinch of salt and pepper over the ingredients. Adjust to taste.

8. **Drizzle Dressing:**
   - Drizzle Greek yogurt-based dressing or lime crema over the wrap for a creamy and tangy touch.

9. **Optional Fresh Cilantro (Optional):**
   - If you enjoy cilantro, sprinkle fresh cilantro leaves over the ingredients for added freshness.

10. **Fold and Roll:**
    - Carefully fold and roll the wrap, securing the ingredients inside.

11. **Slice and Serve:**

- Slice the Shrimp and Avocado Wrap in half diagonally or leave it whole. Serve immediately.

12. **Enjoy Your Flavorful Wrap:**
   - Savor the delightful combination of succulent shrimp, creamy avocado, and crisp veggies in this Shrimp and Avocado Wrap.

Feel free to customize your wrap by adding ingredients like shredded cheese, sliced red onion, or a squeeze of lime for extra flavor. This recipe offers a delicious and protein-packed option during the breast cancer journey.

Vegetable and Lentil Soup

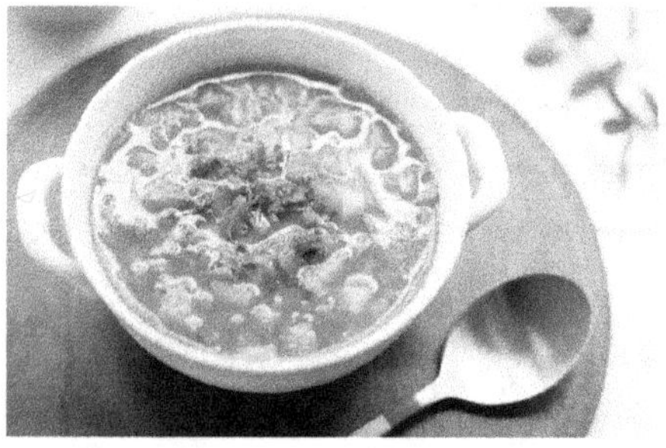

Certainly! Here's a hearty and nutritious recipe for Vegetable and Lentil Soup:

Ingredients:
- One cup rinsed and drained dried lentils, either brown or green

- 1 onion, finely chopped
- 2 carrots, peeled and diced
- 2 celery stalks, diced
- 3 cloves garlic, minced
- 1 can (14 oz) diced tomatoes
- 1 zucchini, diced
- 1 cup green beans, chopped
- 6 cups vegetable broth
- 1 teaspoon dried thyme
- 1 teaspoon dried oregano
- 1 bay leaf
- Salt and pepper to taste
- Olive oil for sautéing
- Fresh parsley for garnish

Instructions:

1. **Sauté Vegetables:**
   - Olive oil should be heated over medium heat in a big pot. Sauté onions, carrots, and celery until softened.

2. **Add Garlic and Herbs:**
   - Add minced garlic, dried thyme, dried oregano, and a bay leaf. Stir for about a minute until fragrant.

3. **Add Lentils and Broth:**
   - Add rinsed lentils, diced tomatoes, zucchini, and green beans to the pot. Pour in vegetable broth.

4. **Season and Simmer:**

- To taste, add salt and pepper for seasoning.
Bring the soup to a boil, then reduce heat to low,
cover, and let it simmer for about 20-25 minutes or
until lentils and vegetables are tender.

5. **Adjust Seasoning:**
   - Taste and adjust the seasoning if needed.
Remove the bay leaf.

6. **Serve Hot:**
   - Ladle the Vegetable and Lentil Soup into bowls.

7. **Garnish with Fresh Parsley:**
   - For a pop of freshness, add some chopped
fresh parsley as a garnish.

8. **Optional Additions (Optional):**
   - Customize your soup by adding a squeeze of
lemon juice or a drizzle of olive oil just before
serving.

9. **Enjoy Your Nourishing Soup:**
   - Enjoy this wholesome Vegetable and Lentil
Soup, packed with fiber, protein, and a variety of
vegetables.

This soup not only provides a comforting and
flavorful meal but also offers a balance of essential
nutrients, making it a nourishing choice during the
breast cancer journey.

Turkey and Hummus Whole Wheat Wrap

Certainly! Here's a delicious recipe for a Turkey and Hummus Whole Wheat Wrap:

Ingredients:
- Whole wheat wrap or tortilla
- Sliced turkey breast
- Hummus
- Spinach leaves
- Sliced cucumbers
- Tomatoes, thinly sliced
- Greek yogurt-based dressing or tzatziki sauce
- Salt and pepper to taste

Instructions:

1. **Prepare Ingredients:**
   - Lay out the whole wheat wrap on a flat surface.

2. **Spread Hummus:**
   - Spread a generous layer of hummus over the entire surface of the wrap.

3. **Layer Turkey Slices:**
   - Arrange slices of turkey breast evenly over the hummus.

4. **Add Spinach Leaves:**

- Place fresh spinach leaves over the turkey slices.

5. **Top with Cucumbers and Tomatoes:**
   - Add sliced cucumbers and thinly sliced tomatoes on top of the spinach.

6. **Season with Salt and Pepper:**
   - Sprinkle a pinch of salt and pepper over the ingredients. Adjust to taste.

7. **Drizzle Dressing or Tzatziki:**
   - Drizzle Greek yogurt-based dressing or tzatziki sauce over the wrap for a creamy and tangy touch.

8. **Optional Extras (Optional):**
   - If you like, you can add extras like red onion slices, feta cheese, or Kalamata olives for extra flavor.

9. **Fold and Roll:**
   - Carefully fold and roll the wrap, securing the ingredients inside.

10. **Slice and Serve:**
   - Slice the Turkey and Hummus Whole Wheat Wrap in half diagonally or leave it whole. Serve immediately.

11. **Enjoy Your Flavorful Wrap:**

- Enjoy the delightful combination of lean turkey, creamy hummus, and crisp veggies in this Turkey and Hummus Whole Wheat Wrap.

Feel free to customize your wrap with your favorite vegetables or additional toppings. This recipe offers a tasty and protein-packed option during the breast cancer journey.

Feel free to adapt these recipes based on your dietary preferences and restrictions. These lunch ideas aim to provide a mix of proteins, healthy fats, whole grains, and a variety of vegetables to support a balanced and nourishing meal during the breast cancer journey.

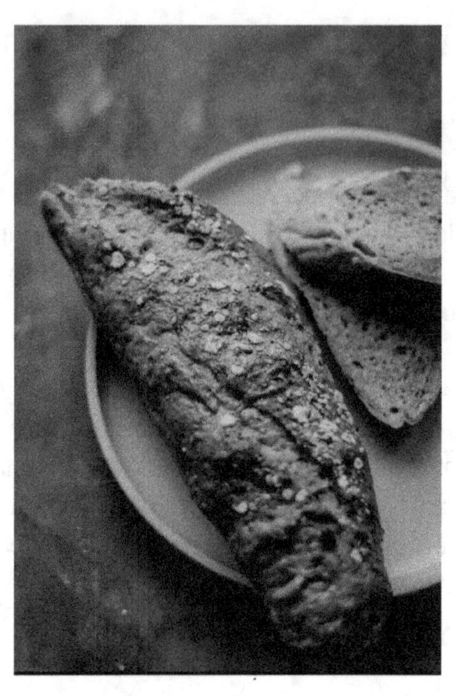

CHAPTER FOUR

SATISFYING DINNER

Certainly! Here are 10 satisfying dinner recipes with detailed instructions, keeping in mind considerations for individuals dealing with breast cancer

Grilled Lemon Herb Chicken

Certainly! Here's a detailed recipe for Grilled Lemon Herb Chicken:

Ingredients:
- 4 boneless, skinless chicken breasts
- 1/4 cup olive oil
- 3 tablespoons fresh lemon juice
- 2 cloves garlic, minced
- 1 teaspoon dried oregano
- 1 teaspoon dried thyme
- 1 teaspoon dried rosemary
- Salt and pepper to taste
- Lemon slices for garnish

Instructions:

1. **Prepare the Marinade:**

- In a bowl, whisk together olive oil, fresh lemon juice, minced garlic, dried oregano, dried thyme, dried rosemary, salt, and pepper.

2. **Marinate the Chicken:**
   - Put the chicken breasts in a shallow dish or resealable plastic bag. Make sure every piece of chicken is covered with marinade by pouring it over it. Refrigerate for a minimum of 30 minutes or for up to 4 hours after sealing the bag or covering the dish.

3. **Preheat the Grill:**
   - Preheat your grill to medium-high heat.

4. **Remove Chicken from Marinade:**
   - Take the chicken out of the refrigerator and let it come to room temperature for about 15 minutes. Take the chicken out of the marinade and let any extra run off.

5. **Grill the Chicken:**
   - Place the chicken on the preheated grill. Grill for approximately 6-8 minutes per side, or until the internal temperature reaches 165°F (74°C) and the chicken is no longer pink in the center.

6. **Baste with Marinade (Optional):**
   - Optionally, baste the chicken with the reserved marinade during the last few minutes of grilling for extra flavor.

7. **Let it Rest:**
   - Remove the grilled lemon herb chicken from the grill and let it rest for a few minutes before serving.

8. **Garnish and Serve:**
   - Add some fresh lemon slices as a garnish for the chicken. Serve the grilled lemon herb chicken hot.

9. **Pairing Suggestion:**
   - Serve with a side of roasted vegetables, quinoa, or a fresh green salad for a complete and satisfying meal.

10. **Enjoy Your Grilled Delight:**
   - Enjoy the deliciously grilled Lemon Herb Chicken, infused with citrusy flavors and aromatic herbs.

This recipe provides a perfect balance of citrus and herbs, creating a flavorful and tender grilled chicken. It's a delightful and healthy option for a satisfying dinner during the breast cancer journey.

Vegetarian Stuffed Bell Peppers

Certainly! Here's a detailed recipe for Vegetarian Stuffed Bell Peppers:

Ingredients:
- 4 large bell peppers, halved and seeds removed

- 1 cup cooked quinoa
- One can (15 oz) of rinsed and drained black beans
- One cup of fresh, frozen, or canned corn kernels
- 1 cup diced tomatoes
- One cup of shredded cheese, either Mexican blend or cheddar
- 1 teaspoon ground cumin
- 1 teaspoon chili powder
- 1/2 teaspoon garlic powder
- Salt and pepper to taste
- Salsa and sour cream for serving (optional)
- Fresh cilantro for garnish (optional)

Instructions:

1. **Preheat the Oven:**
   - Set the oven temperature to 375°F, or 190°C.

2. **Prepare Bell Peppers:**
   - Cut the bell peppers in half lengthwise, removing seeds and membranes. Place them in a baking dish.

3. **Cook Quinoa:**
   - Cook quinoa according to package instructions.

4. **Prepare Filling:**
   - In a large mixing bowl, combine cooked quinoa, black beans, corn, diced tomatoes, shredded cheese, ground cumin, chili powder, garlic powder,

salt, and pepper. Blend thoroughly until all components are uniformly blended.

5. **Stuff Bell Peppers:**
   - Spoon the quinoa mixture into each bell pepper half, pressing down gently to pack the filling.

6. **Cover and Bake:**
   - Cover the baking dish with aluminum foil. Bake the bell peppers for 25 to 30 minutes, or until they are soft, in a preheated oven.

7. **Optional Cheese Topping (Optional):**
   - If you prefer, remove the foil during the last 5-10 minutes of baking and sprinkle additional cheese on top for a golden finish.

8. **Check Doneness:**
   - Check for doneness by inserting a fork into the bell peppers; they should be tender but not mushy.

9. **Garnish and Serve:**
   - Take out of the oven and allow the filled bell peppers to cool down a little. Garnish with fresh cilantro if desired.

10. **Serve with Sides:**
    - Serve the Vegetarian Stuffed Bell Peppers with salsa, sour cream, or any preferred sides.

11. **Enjoy Your Flavorful Stuffed Peppers:**

    - Enjoy these nutritious and flavorful Vegetarian Stuffed Bell Peppers as a wholesome and satisfying meal.

Feel free to customize the filling with additional vegetables or spices based on your preferences. This recipe offers a delicious and protein-packed option for a vegetarian dinner during the breast cancer journey.

Salmon and Asparagus Foil Packets

Certainly! Here's a detailed recipe for Salmon and Asparagus Foil Packets:

Ingredients:
- 4 salmon fillets
- 1 bunch asparagus, trimmed
- 2 tablespoons olive oil
- 2 cloves garlic, minced
- 1 lemon, thinly sliced
- Fresh dill, chopped
- Salt and pepper to taste
- Optional: Lemon wedges for serving

Instructions:

1. **Preheat the Oven:**
   - Set the oven temperature to 400°F, or 200°C.

2. **Prepare Foil Packets:**

   - Tear off four sheets of aluminum foil, each large
enough to wrap a salmon fillet and asparagus.
Place one salmon fillet and a handful of trimmed
asparagus on each foil sheet.

3. **Season with Olive Oil and Garlic:**
   - Drizzle olive oil over each salmon fillet and
asparagus bunch. Sprinkle minced garlic evenly
over the salmon and vegetables.

4. **Add Lemon Slices:**
   - Place a couple of lemon slices on top of each
salmon fillet. The lemon will infuse the salmon with
citrus flavor.

5. **Season with Herbs and Spices:**
   - Season each foil packet with salt, pepper, and
freshly chopped dill to taste.

6. **Fold and Seal Packets:**
   - Carefully fold the sides of the foil over the
salmon and vegetables, creating a sealed packet.
Ensure there are no gaps for steam to escape.

7. **Bake in the Oven:**
   - Place the foil packets on a baking sheet and
bake in the preheated oven for approximately 15-20
minutes or until the salmon is cooked through and
flakes easily with a fork.

8. **Check Doneness:**

- Check the doneness of the salmon by opening one packet and testing the fish with a fork. It should be opaque and flaky.

9. **Serve Hot:**
   - Carefully open the foil packets, transfer the salmon and asparagus to plates, and drizzle with any juices from the packets.

10. **Garnish and Serve:**
   - Garnish with additional fresh dill and serve hot. Serve with lemon slices on the side, if desired.

11. **Enjoy Your Flavorful Foil Packets:**
   - Enjoy this delicious and hassle-free Salmon and Asparagus Foil Packets dish, perfect for a quick and healthy dinner.

This recipe ensures a moist and flavorful salmon preparation with the added benefit of minimal cleanup. It's a delightful option during the breast cancer journey, offering a balance of omega-3 fatty acids and nutritious asparagus.

Mushroom and Spinach Risotto

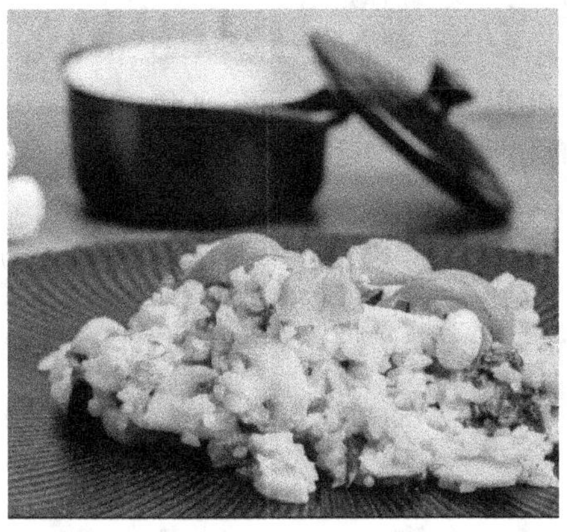

Certainly! Here's a detailed recipe for Mushroom and Spinach Risotto:

Ingredients:
- 1 1/2 cups Arborio rice
- 1/2 cup dry white wine (optional)
- 1 onion, finely chopped
- 2 cloves garlic, minced
- Eight ounces of chopped button or cremini mushrooms
- 3 cups baby spinach, chopped
- 4 cups vegetable broth, kept warm
- 1/2 cup Parmesan cheese, grated
- 2 tablespoons butter
- 2 tablespoons olive oil
- Salt and pepper to taste
- Fresh parsley for garnish

Instructions:

1. **Prepare Mushrooms:**
   - Heat one tablespoon of olive oil in a large skillet. Sliced mushrooms should be added and sautéed until they release moisture and turn golden brown. Set aside.

2. **Sauté Onion and Garlic:**
   - One more tablespoon of olive oil should be added to the same skillet. Minced garlic and diced onion should be sautéed till tender.

3. **Toast Arborio Rice:**
   - Add Arborio rice to the skillet and cook, stirring, until the rice is lightly toasted.

4. **Deglaze with Wine (Optional):**
   - Pour in the white wine, if using, and cook until it's mostly evaporated. If not using wine, proceed to the next step.

5. **Add Broth Gradually:**
   - Begin adding warm vegetable broth, one ladle at a time, stirring frequently. After a while, let the liquid absorb before adding another ladle. Continue this process until the rice is creamy and cooked to al dente texture.

6. **Incorporate Mushrooms and Spinach:**
   - Stir in the sautéed mushrooms and chopped spinach during the last few minutes of cooking until the spinach wilts.

7. **Finish with Butter and Parmesan:**
   - After the rice is cooked, take the skillet off the burner. Stir in butter and grated Parmesan cheese. Season to taste with salt and pepper.

8. **Check Consistency:**
   - If needed, add a bit more warm broth or hot water to achieve the desired creamy consistency.

9. **Garnish and Serve:**
   - Garnish the Mushroom and Spinach Risotto with fresh parsley. Serve hot.

10. **Enjoy Your Creamy Risotto:**
   - Indulge in this creamy and flavorful Mushroom and Spinach Risotto, a comforting dish with a perfect balance of earthy mushrooms and vibrant spinach.

This risotto is not only delicious but also provides a comforting and nutritious option during the breast cancer journey. Adapt the cheese and seasoning to your personal tastes.

Chickpea and Vegetable Stir-Fry

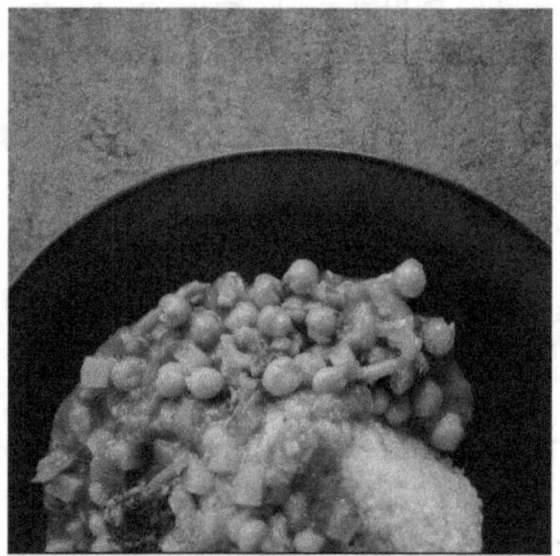

Certainly! Here's a detailed recipe for Chickpea and Vegetable Stir-Fry:

Ingredients:
- 2 cans (15 oz each) chickpeas, drained and rinsed
- 2 cups broccoli florets
- 1 red bell pepper, thinly sliced
- 1 yellow bell pepper, thinly sliced
- 1 carrot, julienned
- 1 zucchini, sliced
- 4 green onions, sliced
- 3 cloves garlic, minced
- 1 tablespoon ginger, grated
- 1/4 cup low-sodium soy sauce
- 2 tablespoons sesame oil
- 1 tablespoon rice vinegar
- 1 tablespoon honey or maple syrup

- 1 tablespoon cornstarch (optional, for thickening)
- 2 tablespoons vegetable oil for stir-frying
- Sesame seeds for garnish (optional)
- Cooked brown rice or quinoa for serving

Instructions:

1. **Prepare Chickpeas:**
   - Rinse and drain chickpeas. Using a paper towel, pat them dry to absorb any remaining moisture.

2. **Mix Stir-Fry Sauce:**
   - In a small bowl, whisk together soy sauce, sesame oil, rice vinegar, and honey (or maple syrup). If you prefer a thicker sauce, mix in cornstarch.

3. **Sauté Chickpeas:**
   - Vegetable oil should be heated over medium-high heat in a large wok or skillet. Add chickpeas and stir-fry for 4-5 minutes until they start to turn golden brown. Remove chickpeas from the wok and set aside.

4. **Stir-Fry Vegetables:**
   - If necessary, add a little extra oil to the same wok. Sauté garlic and ginger until fragrant. Add broccoli, bell peppers, carrot, and zucchini. Sauté the veggies for five to seven minutes, or until they are crisp-tender.

5. **Combine Chickpeas and Sauce:**

- Return the sautéed chickpeas to the wok. Pour the stir-fry sauce over the chickpeas and vegetables. Toss everything together to coat evenly.

6. **Add Green Onions:**
   - Stir in sliced green onions during the last minute of cooking, allowing them to stay fresh and vibrant.

7. **Check Seasoning:**
   - Taste and adjust the seasoning if needed. You can add more soy sauce or honey according to your taste.

8. **Serve Over Rice or Quinoa:**
   - Serve the Chickpea and Vegetable Stir-Fry over cooked brown rice or quinoa.

9. **Garnish and Enjoy:**
   - Garnish with sesame seeds if desired. Enjoy your flavorful and nutritious stir-fry!

This Chickpea and Vegetable Stir-Fry offers a balance of protein, fiber, and vibrant vegetables. It's a delicious and wholesome option during the breast cancer journey. Adjust the vegetable selection based on your preferences.

Eggplant Parmesan

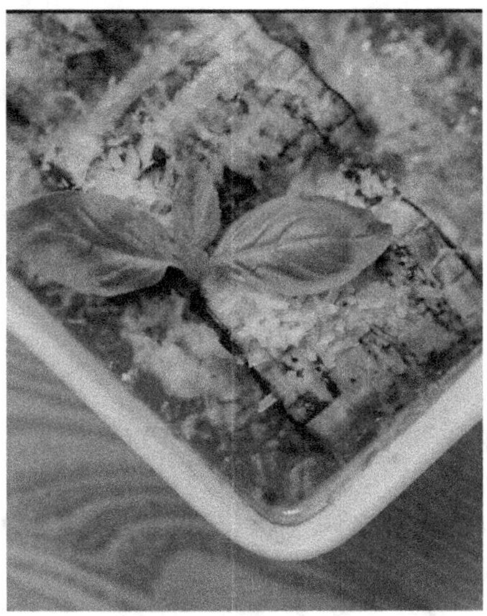

Certainly! Here's a detailed recipe for Eggplant
Parmesan:

Eggplant Parmesan

Ingredients:

- 2 large eggplants, sliced into 1/2-inch rounds
- Salt for sprinkling
- 2 cups all-purpose flour (for dredging)
- 3 large eggs, beaten
- 2 cups Italian-style breadcrumbs
- 1 cup grated Parmesan cheese
- 2 cups marinara sauce
- 2 cups shredded mozzarella cheese

- Garnish with fresh parsley or basil, if desired.

Instructions:

1. **Prepare Eggplant Slices:**
   - Lay the eggplant slices on a paper towel-lined surface. Sprinkle salt on each slice to draw out excess moisture. Let them sit for about 30 minutes, then pat dry with paper towels.

2. **Set Up Dredging Station:**
   - Set up a dredging station with three shallow dishes: one with flour, one with beaten eggs, and one with a mixture of breadcrumbs and grated Parmesan.

3. **Dredge Eggplant Slices:**
   - Dredge each eggplant slice first in the flour, shaking off excess, then dip into the beaten eggs, and coat thoroughly with the breadcrumb-Parmesan mixture.

4. **Preheat Oven:**
   - Set the oven temperature to 375°F, or 190°C.

5. **Bake Eggplant:**
   - Arrange the coated eggplant slices onto a parchment paper-lined baking sheet. Bake in the preheated oven for about 15-20 minutes or until they are golden brown. Flip halfway through the baking time for even browning.

6. **Layer with Marinara and Cheese:**
   - Apply a thin layer of marinara sauce to a baking dish. Place slices of baked eggplant on top in a layer. Cover with more marinara sauce and sprinkle with shredded mozzarella.

7. **Repeat Layering:**
   - Repeat the layering process until all the eggplant slices are used, finishing with a generous layer of marinara and shredded mozzarella on top.

8. **Bake Until Bubbly:**
   - Bake the Eggplant Parmesan in the oven for 25-30 minutes or until the cheese is melted and bubbly, and the edges are golden brown.

9. **Check Doneness:**
   - Check the doneness by inserting a knife into the center; it should go through easily.

10. **Garnish and Serve:**
   - If desired, add some fresh parsley or basil as a garnish. Before serving, let it rest for a few minutes.

11. **Enjoy Your Cheesy Eggplant Parmesan:**
   - Serve the Eggplant Parmesan hot, and enjoy the layers of crispy eggplant, marinara sauce, and gooey melted cheese.

This classic Eggplant Parmesan recipe offers a delicious and satisfying dish, perfect for a comforting dinner during the breast cancer journey.

Adjust the seasoning and cheese quantities according to your preferences.

Quinoa and Black Bean Burrito Bowl

Certainly! Here's a detailed recipe for Quinoa and Black Bean Burrito Bowl:

Ingredients:

- 1 cup quinoa, rinsed
- 2 cups water
- One can (15 oz) of rinsed and drained black beans
- One cup of fresh, frozen, or canned corn kernels
- 1 cup cherry tomatoes, halved
- 1 avocado, diced
- 1/2 red onion, finely diced
- 1 cup shredded lettuce or cabbage
- 1/4 cup fresh cilantro, chopped
- Lime wedges for serving
- Optional: Salsa, Greek yogurt, or sour cream for topping
- Salt and pepper to taste

For the Dressing:

- 2 tablespoons olive oil
- 2 tablespoons lime juice
- 1 teaspoon ground cumin

- 1 teaspoon chili powder
- Salt and pepper to taste

Instructions:

1. **Cook Quinoa:**
   - In a medium saucepan, combine quinoa and water. After bringing to a boil, lower the heat to a simmer, cover, and cook the quinoa for 15 to 20 minutes, or until it is tender and the water has been absorbed.

2. **Prepare Black Beans:**
   - In a small saucepan, heat black beans over medium heat until warmed. Adjust the seasoning with salt and pepper to taste.

3. **Make the Dressing:**
   - In a small bowl, whisk together olive oil, lime juice, ground cumin, chili powder, salt, and pepper. Set aside.

4. **Assemble the Burrito Bowl:**
   - In serving bowls, layer cooked quinoa, black beans, corn, cherry tomatoes, diced avocado, red onion, shredded lettuce or cabbage, and chopped cilantro.

5. **Drizzle with Dressing:**
   - Drizzle the prepared dressing over the burrito bowl ingredients.

6. **Top with Optional Ingredients:**
   - Add additional toppings like salsa, Greek yogurt, or sour cream if desired.

7. **Squeeze Lime Wedges:**
   - Squeeze lime wedges over the bowl for an extra burst of freshness.

8. **Toss Gently:**
   - Gently toss the ingredients in each bowl to distribute the flavors and dressing evenly.

9. **Adjust Seasoning:**
   - Taste and adjust seasoning as needed.

10. **Serve and Enjoy:**
   - Serve the Quinoa and Black Bean Burrito Bowls immediately and enjoy this wholesome and flavorful meal.

This burrito bowl provides a balance of protein, fiber, and essential nutrients, making it a delicious and nourishing option during the breast cancer journey. Customize the toppings based on your preferences for a personalized touch.

Teriyaki Glazed Salmon with Sesame Broccoli

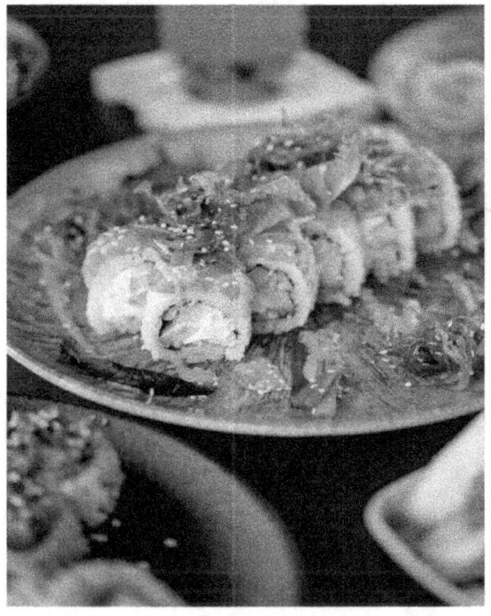

Certainly! Here's a detailed recipe for Teriyaki Glazed Salmon with Sesame Broccoli:

Ingredients:

For Teriyaki Glazed Salmon:

- 4 salmon fillets
- 1/4 cup soy sauce
- 2 tablespoons honey
- 2 tablespoons rice vinegar
- 1 tablespoon sesame oil
- 2 cloves garlic, minced
- 1 teaspoon ginger, grated

- Sesame seeds for garnish (optional)
- Sliced green onions for garnish (optional)

For Sesame Broccoli:

- 4 cups broccoli florets
- 1 tablespoon sesame oil
- 1 tablespoon soy sauce
- 1 tablespoon sesame seeds

Instructions:

For Teriyaki Glazed Salmon:

1. **Prepare the Teriyaki Glaze:**
   - In a bowl, whisk together soy sauce, honey, rice vinegar, sesame oil, minced garlic, and grated ginger to create the teriyaki glaze.

2. **Marinate Salmon:**
   - Place the salmon fillets in a shallow dish and pour half of the teriyaki glaze over them. Allow them to marinate for at least 15-30 minutes.

3. **Preheat Oven:**
   - Set the oven temperature to 400°F, or 200°C.

4. **Bake Salmon:**
   - The salmon fillets should be marinated and placed on a parchment paper-lined baking sheet. Bake the salmon for 12 to 15 minutes, or until it is

cooked through and flake readily, in an oven that
has been warmed.

5. **Brush with Glaze:**
   - During the last few minutes of baking, brush the
salmon with the remaining teriyaki glaze for extra
flavor.

6. **Garnish:**
   - Garnish the baked salmon with sesame seeds
and sliced green onions if desired.

For Sesame Broccoli:

1. **Steam Broccoli:**
   - Broccoli florets should be steamed until they are
crisp-tender. You can steam them on the stovetop
or use a microwave-safe steamer.

2. **Sauté in Sesame Oil:**
   - Heat the sesame oil in a pan over medium heat.
Add the steamed broccoli to the pan.

3. **Add Soy Sauce and Sesame Seeds:**
   - Drizzle soy sauce over the broccoli and sprinkle
sesame seeds. Toss the broccoli until it's well
coated in the sesame-soy mixture.

4. **Serve Together:**
   - Serve the Teriyaki Glazed Salmon fillets
alongside the Sesame Broccoli.

5. **Enjoy Your Flavorful Dish:**
   - Enjoy this delicious and balanced Teriyaki Glazed Salmon with Sesame Broccoli, providing a tasty combination of sweet and savory flavors.

This recipe offers a delightful and nutritious option during the breast cancer journey. To suit your tastes, adjust the ingredients.

Lentil and Vegetable Curry

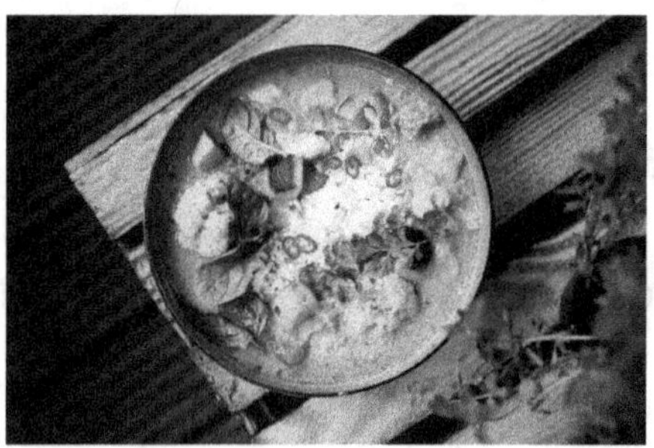

Certainly! Here's a detailed recipe for Lentil and Vegetable Curry:

Ingredients:

- 1 cup dry lentils (red or green), rinsed and drained
- 2 tablespoons vegetable oil
- 1 onion, finely chopped
- 3 cloves garlic, minced
- 1 tablespoon ginger, grated
- 1 bell pepper, diced

- 2 carrots, peeled and sliced
- 1 zucchini, diced
- 1 can (14 oz) diced tomatoes
- 1 can (14 oz) coconut milk
- 2 tablespoons curry powder
- 1 teaspoon ground cumin
- 1 teaspoon ground coriander
- 1/2 teaspoon turmeric
- 1/2 teaspoon cayenne pepper (optional, for heat)
- Salt and pepper to taste
- Fresh cilantro for garnish
- Cooked rice or naan for serving

Instructions:

1. **Cook Lentils:**
   - In a pot, combine lentils with water (follow package instructions) and cook until lentils are tender. Drain any excess water.

2. **Sauté Aromatics:**
   - In a large skillet or pot, heat vegetable oil over medium heat. Add chopped onion and sauté until softened. Add minced garlic and grated ginger, and cook for an additional minute until fragrant.

3. **Add Vegetables:**
   - Add diced bell pepper, sliced carrots, and diced zucchini to the skillet. Sauté until vegetables are slightly softened.

4. **Spice it Up:**

- Add the turmeric, cayenne pepper (if using), ground cumin, ground coriander, and curry powder. Toss to thoroughly coat the veggies with the spice mixture.

5. **Combine with Lentils:**
   - Add the cooked lentils to the skillet and mix with the vegetables and spices.

6. **Pour in Tomatoes and Coconut Milk:**
   - Pour in diced tomatoes (with their juices) and coconut milk. Stir to combine all the ingredients.

7. **Simmer:**
   - Bring the curry to a gentle simmer. Allow the flavors to combine and the vegetables to soften for approximately 15 to 20 minutes of cooking.

8. **Season and Garnish:**
   - Season the lentil and vegetable curry with salt and pepper to taste. Garnish with fresh cilantro.

9. **Serve Over Rice or with Naan:**
   - Serve the curry over cooked rice or with naan bread for a complete and satisfying meal.

10. **Enjoy Your Hearty Lentil Curry:**
    - Enjoy this hearty and flavorful Lentil and Vegetable Curry, rich in protein and vibrant spices.

Feel free to customize the vegetables or adjust the spice levels according to your preferences. This curry provides a comforting and nutritious option during the breast cancer journey.

Spinach and Feta Stuffed Chicken Breast

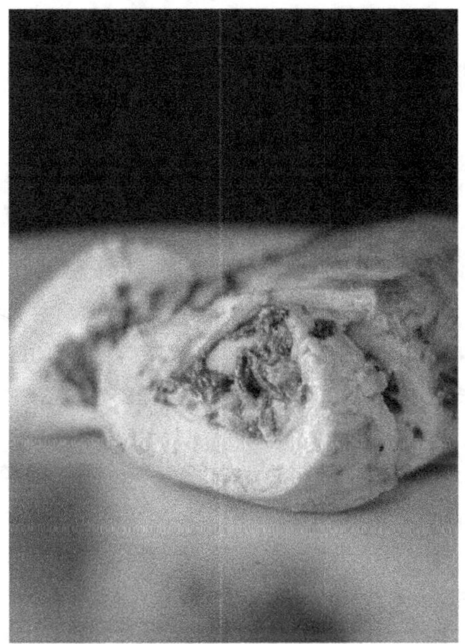

Certainly! Here's a detailed recipe for Spinach and Feta Stuffed Chicken Breast:

Ingredients:

- 4 boneless, skinless chicken breasts
- 2 cups fresh spinach, chopped
- 1/2 cup feta cheese, crumbled

- 1/4 cup sun-dried tomatoes, chopped (optional)
- 2 cloves garlic, minced
- 1 tablespoon olive oil
- 1 teaspoon dried oregano
- Salt and pepper to taste
- Toothpicks or kitchen twine
- Lemon wedges for serving (optional)

Instructions:

1. **Preheat Oven:**
   - Set the oven temperature to 375°F, or 190°C.

2. **Prepare Spinach and Feta Filling:**
   - In a skillet, heat olive oil over medium heat. Add minced garlic and sauté until fragrant. Add chopped spinach and cook until wilted. Remove from heat and let it cool. Once cooled, stir in crumbled feta and chopped sun-dried tomatoes if using. Add salt, pepper, and dried oregano for seasoning.

3. **Butterfly Chicken Breasts:**
   - On a chopping board, place one chicken breast flat. With a sharp knife, cut horizontally through the center, almost to the other side, creating a pocket without cutting all the way through.

4. **Stuff Chicken Breasts:**
   - Stuff each chicken breast with the spinach and feta mixture, pressing the edges to seal. If needed, secure with toothpicks or tie with kitchen twine.

5. **Season Chicken:**
   - Season the outside of each stuffed chicken breast with a bit of salt, pepper, and additional oregano if desired.

6. **Sear Chicken:**
   - In an oven-safe skillet, heat a bit of olive oil over medium-high heat. Sear each stuffed chicken breast for 2-3 minutes on each side until golden brown.

7. **Transfer to Oven:**
   - Transfer the skillet to the preheated oven and bake for 20-25 minutes or until the chicken is cooked through, with no pink in the center.

8. **Check Doneness:**
   - Check the doneness by inserting a meat thermometer into the thickest part of the chicken; it should read 165°F (74°C).

9. **Rest and Serve:**
   - Remove from the oven and let the stuffed chicken breasts rest for a few minutes before serving.

10. **Optional Lemon Wedges:**
   - For a zesty touch, serve with lemon slices on the side.

11. **Enjoy Your Elegant Stuffed Chicken:**

- Enjoy this elegant and flavorful Spinach and Feta Stuffed Chicken Breast as a delicious and protein-packed dish during the breast cancer journey.

Feel free to customize the stuffing with your favorite herbs or additional ingredients. This recipe provides a delightful combination of tender chicken, savory spinach, and creamy feta.

Feel free to adjust the ingredients and portions based on your preferences and dietary needs. These recipes offer a variety of flavors and nutrients for satisfying dinners during the breast cancer journey.

CHAPTER FIVE

SNACKS FOR STRENGTH

Certainly! Here are six snack recipes for strength with detailed instructions, keeping in mind considerations for individuals dealing with breast cancer:

Protein-Packed Energy Bites

Certainly! Here's a detailed recipe for Protein-Packed Energy Bites:

Ingredients:

- 1 cup rolled oats
- 1/2 cup peanut butter
- 1/3 cup honey or maple syrup
- 1/2 cup protein powder
- 1/2 cup dark chocolate chips
- 1 teaspoon vanilla extract
- Pinch of salt

Instructions:

1. **Combine Dry Ingredients:**
   - In a mixing bowl, combine rolled oats, protein powder, and a pinch of salt.

2. **Add Wet Ingredients:**
   - Add peanut butter, honey or maple syrup, dark chocolate chips, and vanilla extract to the dry ingredients.

3. **Mix Well:**
   - Mix the ingredients thoroughly until well combined. The mixture should be sticky and easily moldable.

4. **Chill in the Refrigerator:**
   - Refrigerate the mixture for fifteen to thirty minutes. Chilling helps make it easier to form into balls.

5. **Shape into Bites:**
   - Once chilled, take small portions of the mixture and roll them into bite-sized balls. Use your hands to shape them evenly.

6. **Set in the Fridge:**
   - Place the energy bites on a tray lined with parchment paper and refrigerate for an additional 15-30 minutes to firm up.

7. **Store and Enjoy:**
   - Transfer the protein-packed energy bites to an airtight container. You can Store them in the refrigerator for up to two weeks.

8. **Savor the Energy Bites:**

- Enjoy these delicious and nutritious Protein-Packed Energy Bites as a quick and energizing snack.

These energy bites are not only a convenient snack but also provide a good balance of protein, healthy fats, and carbohydrates, making them a great option for sustained energy during the day. To fit your dietary requirements and taste preferences, modify the components.

Greek Yogurt Parfait with Berries

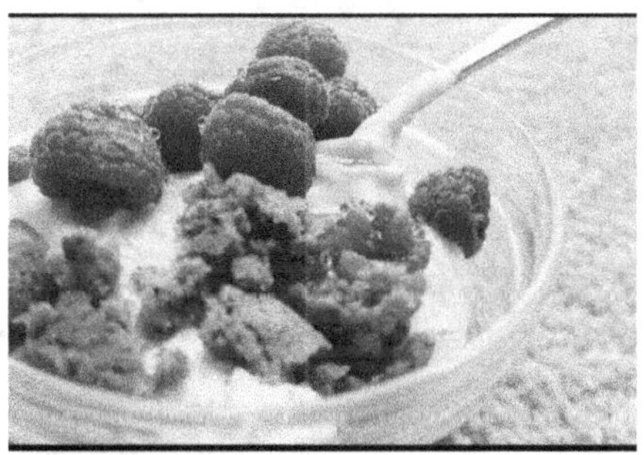

Certainly! Here's a detailed recipe for Greek Yogurt Parfait with Berries:

Ingredients:

- 1 cup Greek yogurt
- 1/2 cup granola
- Half a cup of mixed berries, including raspberries, blueberries, and strawberries
- Honey for drizzling (optional)

Instructions:

1. **Prepare Ingredients:**
   - Gather Greek yogurt, granola, and a mix of fresh berries.

2. **Layer Greek Yogurt:**
   - In a glass or bowl, start by adding a layer of Greek yogurt. Use about a third of the total amount.

3. **Add Granola Layer:**
   - Sprinkle a layer of granola over the Greek yogurt. This adds a crunchy texture and additional nutrients.

4. **Introduce Berry Layer:**
   - Spread some mixed berries over the granola. Ensure an even distribution of different berries for a colorful and flavorful parfait.

5. **Repeat Layers:**
   - Repeat the layering process, starting with Greek yogurt, followed by granola, and then berries until you fill the glass or bowl.

6. **Drizzle with Honey (Optional):**
   - For extra sweetness, you can drizzle honey over the top layer of berries. To suit your tastes, adjust the quantity.

7. **Serve Immediately:**

   - Serve the Greek Yogurt Parfait immediately to enjoy the contrast of creamy yogurt, crunchy granola, and juicy berries.

8. **Customize and Enjoy:**
   - Feel free to customize your parfait by adding nuts, seeds, or a dollop of nut butter for added flavor and nutrition.

This Greek Yogurt Parfait with Berries not only makes for a visually appealing snack but also provides a combination of protein, fiber, and antioxidants. It's a delightful and wholesome option for a quick and nutritious treat.

Hummus and Veggie Sticks

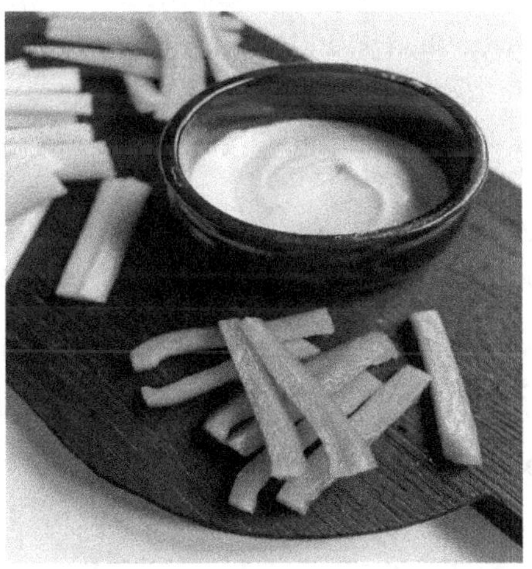

Certainly! Here's a detailed recipe for Hummus and Veggie Sticks:

Ingredients:

- 1 cup hummus (store-bought or homemade)
- Cucumber slices, bell pepper pieces, and carrot sticks for dipping

Instructions:

1. **Prepare Hummus:**
   - If you're making hummus at home, blend chickpeas, tahini, olive oil, lemon juice, garlic, and salt in a food processor until smooth. Adjust ingredients to taste.

2. **Cut Vegetables:**
   - Wash and peel carrots. Cut them into sticks.
   - Wash and slice cucumber into thin rounds or sticks.
   - Wash, seed, and thinly slice bell peppers.

3. **Arrange Vegetables:**
   - Arrange the carrot sticks, cucumber slices, and bell pepper strips on a serving platter.

4. **Serve with Hummus:**
   - Place a bowl of hummus in the center of the platter or in individual dipping bowls.

5. **Dip and Enjoy:**
   - Dip the veggie sticks into the hummus and enjoy a nutritious and satisfying snack.

6. **Optional Garnish:**
   - Optionally, drizzle a little olive oil over the hummus and sprinkle with paprika or chopped fresh herbs for extra flavor and presentation.

7. **Variations:**
   - Feel free to experiment with other veggies like cherry tomatoes, celery sticks, or broccoli florets.

8. **Enjoy a Healthy Snack:**
   - Hummus and Veggie Sticks make for a wholesome and balanced snack, providing a combination of protein, fiber, and vitamins.

This simple and nutritious snack is not only delicious but also a great way to incorporate more vegetables into your diet. Adjust the quantity of hummus and veggies based on your preferences.

Trail Mix Power Bowl

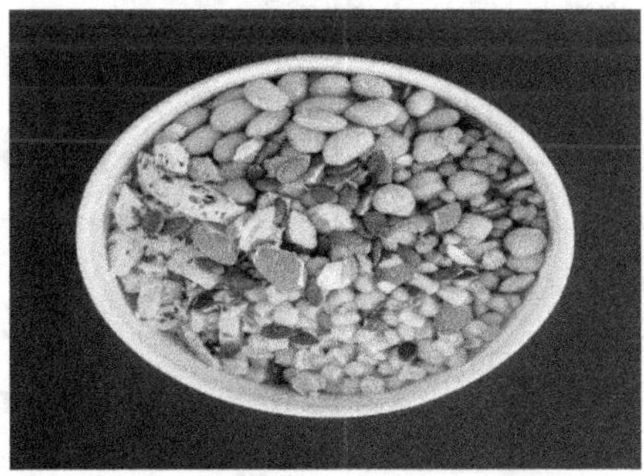

Certainly! Here's a detailed recipe for a Trail Mix Power Bowl:

Ingredients:

- 1/2 cup almonds
- 1/2 cup walnuts
- 1/4 cup pumpkin seeds
- 1/4 cup dried cranberries
- 1/4 cup dark chocolate chunks

Instructions:

1. **Combine Nuts and Seeds:**
   - In a mixing bowl, combine almonds, walnuts, and pumpkin seeds.

2. **Add Dried Fruits:**
   - Mix in dried cranberries to add a sweet and tart flavor to the trail mix.

3. **Include Dark Chocolate Chunks:**
   - Add dark chocolate chunks to the mix for a delightful touch of sweetness.

4. **Mix Thoroughly:**
   - Gently stir all the ingredients until thoroughly blended.

5. **Portion into Serving Bowls:**
   - Portion the trail mix into individual serving bowls or containers.

6. **Optional: Customize the Mix:**

   - Feel free to customize the trail mix by adding your favorite nuts, seeds, or dried fruits.

7. **Serve and Enjoy:**
   - Enjoy the Trail Mix Power Bowl as a convenient and energy-boosting snack.

8. **On-the-Go Option:**
   - Pack individual servings in small containers for a portable snack that can be enjoyed at work, school, or during outdoor activities.

9. **Store in an Airtight Container:**
   - If not consuming immediately, store the trail mix in an airtight container to maintain freshness.

This Trail Mix Power Bowl is not only tasty but also provides a mix of healthy fats, protein, and antioxidants. It's a perfect option for a quick and satisfying snack to keep you energized throughout the day. Adapt the ingredients to suit your dietary requirements and preferences.

Cottage Cheese and Pineapple Cups

Certainly! Here's a detailed recipe for Cottage Cheese and Pineapple Cups:

Ingredients:

- 1 cup cottage cheese

- 1 cup fresh pineapple chunks

Instructions:

1. **Prepare Cottage Cheese:**
   - If using store-bought cottage cheese, simply measure out 1 cup. If making cottage cheese at home, follow your preferred recipe or purchase it from a trusted source.

2. **Cut Fresh Pineapple:**
   - Peel and core a fresh pineapple. Cut it into bite-sized chunks, aiming for about 1 cup.

3. **Assemble Cups:**
   - In serving bowls or cups, layer cottage cheese and fresh pineapple chunks.

4. **Alternate Layers:**
   - Create alternate layers of cottage cheese and pineapple until you fill the cups.

5. **Serve Chilled:**
   - Refrigerate the Cottage Cheese and Pineapple Cups for at least 30 minutes before serving. Chilling enhances the flavors and provides a refreshing element.

6. **Optional Garnish:**
   - Optionally, garnish the cups with a mint leaf or a sprinkle of shredded coconut for added freshness and visual appeal.

7. **Enjoy a Healthy Snack:**
   - Serve these Cottage Cheese and Pineapple Cups as a light and nutritious snack, perfect for a quick pick-me-up.

8. **Customize to Taste:**
   - Feel free to customize the recipe by adding a drizzle of honey or a sprinkle of your favorite nuts for extra flavor and texture.

9. **Healthy and Protein-Rich:**
   - Cottage Cheese and Pineapple Cups provide a balance of protein from cottage cheese and natural sweetness from pineapple, making them a healthy and satisfying snack.

This simple and delightful snack is not only tasty but also a great source of protein and vitamins. Adjust the quantities based on your preferences and enjoy this refreshing combination.

Avocado Toast with Poached Egg

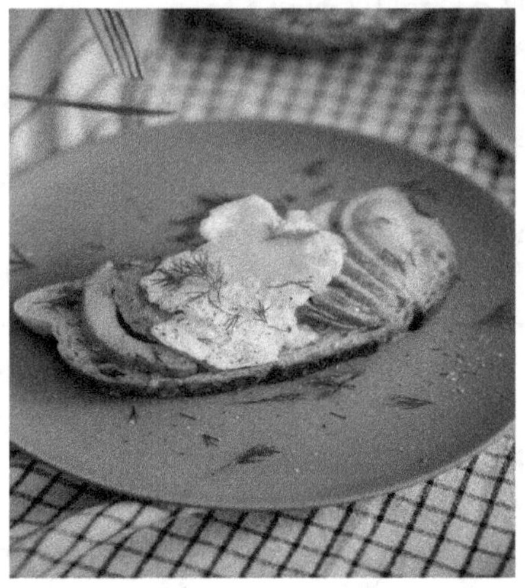

Certainly! Here's a detailed recipe for Avocado Toast with Poached Egg:

Ingredients:

- 1 slice whole-grain bread
- 1/2 ripe avocado
- 1 poached egg
- Salt and pepper to taste
- Optional: Red pepper flakes for a kick

Instructions:

1. **Toast the Bread:**
   - Toast a slice of whole-grain bread to your desired level of crispiness.

2. **Prepare the Avocado:**
   - While the bread is toasting, cut a ripe avocado in half. Scoop out the flesh and mash it with a fork in a bowl.

3. **Spread Avocado on Toast:**
   - On the toasted bread, equally distribute the mashed avocado.

4. **Poach the Egg:**
   - Use your favorite technique to poach an egg. If you're not familiar with poaching eggs, a common method is to simmer an egg in water until the white is set but the yolk remains runny. You can use a poaching pan or follow various online tutorials for poaching eggs.

5. **Place Poached Egg on Avocado Toast:**
   - Carefully place the poached egg on top of the mashed avocado on the toast.

6. **Season with Salt and Pepper:**
   - To taste, add salt and pepper to the poached egg. Adjust the seasoning based on your preference.

7. **Optional: Add Red Pepper Flakes:**
   - For a bit of heat, you can sprinkle red pepper flakes over the poached egg.

8. **Serve Immediately:**

- Serve the Avocado Toast with Poached Egg
immediately while the egg is still warm.

9. **Enjoy a Nutrient-Rich Breakfast:**
   - Enjoy this delicious and nutrient-rich breakfast,
combining the creamy texture of avocado with the
protein and richness of a poached egg.

10. **Variations:**
   - Experiment with additional toppings such as
cherry tomatoes, feta cheese, or a drizzle of
balsamic glaze for added flavor.

This Avocado Toast with Poached Egg is a popular
and satisfying choice for a healthy breakfast or
brunch. It provides a good balance of healthy fats,
protein, and whole grains to kick-start your day.

These snacks are not only delicious but also
packed with nutrients to support strength and
energy during the day. Adjust portions based on
your dietary needs.

CHAPTER SIX

GUILT-FREE DESSERTS

Certainly! Here are five guilt-free dessert recipes with detailed instructions, keeping in mind considerations for individuals dealing with breast cancer:

Berry Yogurt Parfait

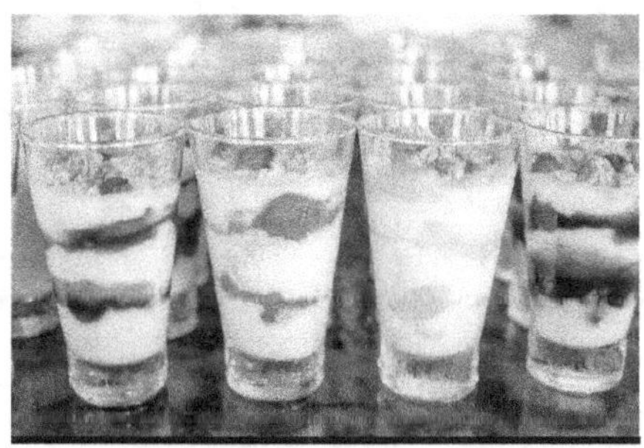

Certainly! Here's a detailed recipe for Berry Yogurt Parfait:

Ingredients:

- 1 cup Greek yogurt (unsweetened)
- Half a cup of mixed berries, including raspberries, blueberries, and strawberries
- One tablespoon of maple syrup or honey (optional)

- 2 tablespoons chopped nuts (almonds, walnuts)

Instructions:

1. **Prepare Ingredients:**
   - Gather Greek yogurt, mixed berries, honey or maple syrup (if using), and chopped nuts.

2. **Layer Greek Yogurt:**
   - In a glass or bowl, start by adding a layer of Greek yogurt. Use about a third of the total amount.

3. **Add Berry Layer:**
   - Add a layer of mixed berries on top of the Greek yogurt. Ensure an even distribution of different berries for a burst of flavors.

4. **Drizzle with Honey (Optional):**
   - If you desire added sweetness, drizzle honey or maple syrup over the berry layer.

5. **Sprinkle Chopped Nuts:**
   - Sprinkle chopped nuts (almonds, walnuts) over the berry layer for added crunch and nutrition.

6. **Repeat Layers:**
   - Repeat the layering process, starting with Greek yogurt, then berries, honey (optional), and chopped nuts.

7. **Garnish with Whole Berries:**

  - Garnish the top layer with a few whole berries
for a visually appealing presentation.

8. **Serve Immediately:**
  - Serve the Berry Yogurt Parfait immediately to
enjoy the contrast of creamy yogurt, sweet berries,
and crunchy nuts.

9. **Customize to Taste:**
  - Feel free to customize your parfait by adding
granola, seeds, or a sprinkle of cinnamon for
additional flavor and texture.

10. **Enjoy Your Guilt-Free Parfait:**
  - Relish this guilt-free and nutritious Berry Yogurt
Parfait as a satisfying snack or a wholesome
dessert.

This simple and vibrant parfait is not only delicious
but also provides a mix of protein, vitamins, and
antioxidants. Adjust the quantities based on your
preferences and dietary needs.

Coconut Date Bites

Certainly! Here's a detailed recipe for Coconut Date
Bites:

Ingredients:

- 1 cup dates, pitted

- 1/2 cup shredded coconut (unsweetened)
- 1/4 cup raw almonds
- 1/4 cup chia seeds
- 1 teaspoon vanilla extract

Instructions:

1. **Prepare Ingredients:**
   - Ensure that the dates are pitted. If not already done, pit the dates before using.

2. **Combine in Food Processor:**
   - In a food processor, combine pitted dates, shredded coconut, raw almonds, chia seeds, and vanilla extract.

3. **Process until Sticky Dough Forms:**
   - Process the ingredients until they come together into a sticky and uniform dough. The mixture should be easily moldable.

4. **Roll into Bites:**
   - To make bite-sized balls, take little parts of the dough and roll them between your palms.

5. **Optional: Coat with Additional Coconut:**
   - If desired, roll the date bites in additional shredded coconut to coat the exterior.

6. **Chill in Refrigerator:**

- Place the date bites on a plate or tray and refrigerate for at least 30 minutes. Chilling helps them firm up.

7. **Serve and Enjoy:**
   - Once chilled, the Coconut Date Bites are ready to be served. Enjoy these delightful and nutritious bites.

8. **Store in Refrigerator:**
   - Store any remaining date bites in an airtight container in the refrigerator for freshness.

9. **Customize as Desired:**
   - Feel free to customize the recipe by adding a touch of cinnamon, a sprinkle of sea salt, or other favorite ingredients.

10. **Enjoy a Healthy Sweet Treat:**
    - These Coconut Date Bites provide a naturally sweet and satisfying treat without added sugars. They are rich in fiber, healthy fats, and vitamins.

These Coconut Date Bites make for a perfect guilt-free snack or a naturally sweet dessert. Adjust the ingredients according to your taste preferences and dietary needs.

Baked Cinnamon Apples

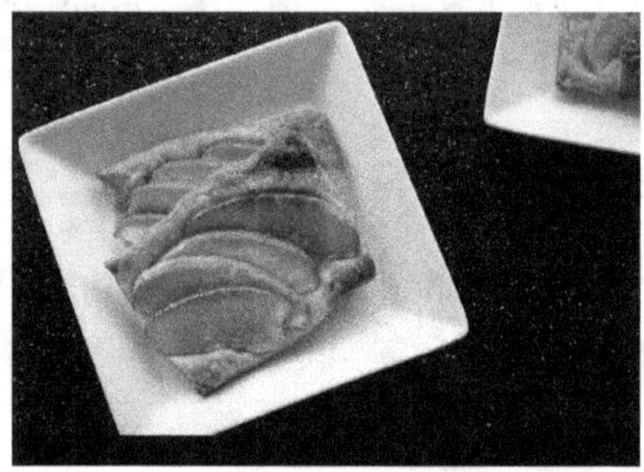

Certainly! Here's a detailed recipe for Baked
Cinnamon Apples:

Ingredients:

- 4 apples, cored and sliced
- 1 teaspoon cinnamon
- 2 tablespoons chopped walnuts
- 1 tablespoon coconut oil (melted)

Instructions:

1. **Preheat the Oven:**
   - Set the oven temperature to 375°F, or 190°C.

2. **Prepare Apples:**
   - Wash, core, and slice the apples. Keep the skin
on for more nutrients and fiber.

3. **Toss with Cinnamon:**

   - In a mixing bowl, toss the apple slices with
cinnamon until they are evenly coated. The
cinnamon adds warmth and flavor.

4. **Add Chopped Walnuts:**
   - Add chopped walnuts to the bowl and gently
toss with the apple slices. Walnuts provide a
delightful crunch and additional nutritional benefits.

5. **Coat with Coconut Oil:**
   - Drizzle melted coconut oil over the apple
mixture. Ensure all slices are coated evenly.

6. **Mix Well:**
   - Mix the ingredients well to ensure the apples are
coated with the cinnamon, walnuts, and coconut oil.

7. **Bake in Oven:**
   - Spread the apple mixture evenly on a baking
sheet lined with parchment paper.

8. **Bake Until Tender:**
   - Bake in the preheated oven for 20-25 minutes or
until the apples are tender. Keep a close eye on
them to prevent overcooking.

9. **Optional: Serve Warm:**
   - Once baked, you can serve the cinnamon
apples warm. They make a delicious and
comforting dessert or snack.

10. **Enjoy a Healthy Dessert:**

- Enjoy these Baked Cinnamon Apples as a healthier alternative to traditional desserts. They are naturally sweet and provide a dose of fiber and nutrients.

11. **Optional Additions:**
   - Feel free to experiment by adding a drizzle of honey or maple syrup for extra sweetness or a sprinkle of nutmeg for additional warmth.

12. **Store Any Leftovers:**
   - If you have any leftovers, put them in the fridge in an airtight container. You can eat them cold or warm.

These Baked Cinnamon Apples offer a delightful combination of sweetness and warmth without added sugars. They are a great way to enjoy a comforting dessert with the natural goodness of apples.

Chia Seed Pudding with Mango

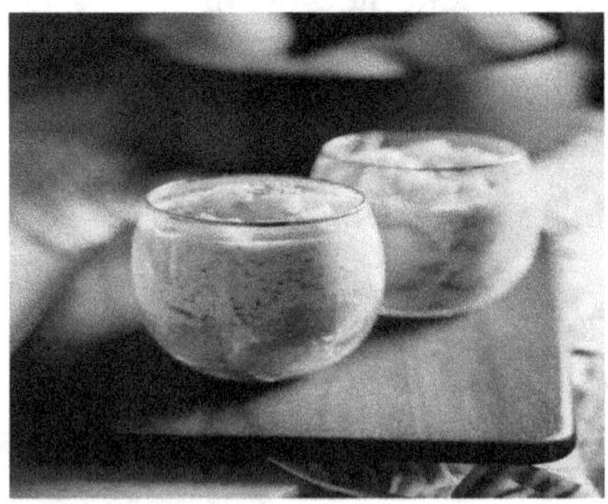

Certainly! Here's a detailed recipe for Chia Seed Pudding with Mango:

Ingredients:

- 3 tablespoons chia seeds
- 1 cup coconut milk (unsweetened)
- 1 tablespoon honey or maple syrup
- 1/2 teaspoon vanilla extract
- 1 ripe mango, diced

Instructions:

1. **Combine Chia Seeds and Coconut Milk:**
   - In a jar or bowl, combine chia seeds, coconut milk, honey or maple syrup, and vanilla extract.

2. **Stir Well:**
   - Stir the mixture thoroughly to ensure that the chia seeds are well distributed and don't clump together.

3. **Refrigerate:**
   - Cover the jar or bowl and refrigerate the chia seed mixture for at least 4 hours or overnight. In doing so, the liquid can be absorbed by the chia seeds, creating a pudding-like consistency.

4. **Stir Again:**

- After the initial refrigeration, give the chia seed pudding a good stir to break up any clumps that may have formed.

5. **Layer with Diced Mango:**
   - In serving glasses or bowls, layer the chia seed pudding with diced mango. You can alternate layers or create a bottom layer of pudding topped with mango.

6. **Repeat Layers:**
   - Continue layering until you've used up all the chia seed pudding and mango.

7. **Top with Additional Mango:**
   - Finish by topping the Chia Seed Pudding with additional diced mango for a fresh and vibrant touch.

8. **Optional: Drizzle with Honey:**
   - Optionally, drizzle a bit of honey over the top for added sweetness.

9. **Serve Chilled:**
   - Serve the Chia Seed Pudding with Mango chilled and enjoy the delightful combination of creamy pudding and sweet mango.

10. **Customize to Taste:**
   - Feel free to experiment with toppings such as shredded coconut, nuts, or a sprinkle of cinnamon to add extra flavor and texture.

11. **Enjoy a Nutrient-Rich Dessert:**
   - This Chia Seed Pudding with Mango is not only a delicious dessert but also a nutritious one, packed with omega-3 fatty acids, fiber, and vitamins.

You are welcome to modify the sweetness and consistency to suit your tastes. This dessert is perfect for a healthy and satisfying treat.

Frozen Banana Bites

Certainly! Here's a detailed recipe for Frozen Banana Bites:

Ingredients:

- 2 bananas, peeled and sliced
- 1/4 cup dark chocolate, melted
- 2 tablespoons shredded coconut (unsweetened)

Instructions:

1. **Prepare Bananas:**
   - After peeling, cut the bananas into little rounds. Ensure the rounds are not too thick for easier handling.

2. **Melt Dark Chocolate:**

- In a microwave-safe bowl or using a double boiler, melt the dark chocolate until smooth. Stir well to ensure a silky consistency.

3. **Dip Banana Slices:**
   - Dip each banana slice into the melted dark chocolate, ensuring that it's evenly coated. You can use a fork or toothpick for easy dipping.

4. **Place on Parchment Paper:**
   - Place the chocolate-coated banana slices on a parchment paper-lined tray. Ensure they are not touching each other to prevent sticking.

5. **Sprinkle with Shredded Coconut:**
   - While the chocolate is still wet, sprinkle shredded coconut over the banana slices. This adds a delightful texture and flavor.

6. **Freeze Until Solid:**
   - Transfer the tray to the freezer and let the banana bites freeze until solid. This usually takes about 2-3 hours.

7. **Store in Freezer Bag or Container:**
   - Once frozen, transfer the banana bites into a freezer bag or airtight container for convenient storage.

8. **Serve and Enjoy:**

   - Serve the Frozen Banana Bites straight from the
freezer and enjoy the perfect blend of creamy
banana and rich dark chocolate.

9. **Optional: Experiment with Toppings:**
   - Feel free to experiment with additional toppings
like chopped nuts, chia seeds, or a drizzle of
almond butter for added variety.

10. **Savor a Healthy Sweet Treat:**
   - These Frozen Banana Bites make for a
guilt-free and refreshing sweet treat. They are not
only delicious but also a source of natural sugars,
potassium, and antioxidants.

11. **Customize to Taste:**
   - Adjust the thickness of the banana slices and
the amount of chocolate and coconut based on
your preferences.

These Frozen Banana Bites are a great alternative
to traditional ice cream treats and are perfect for a
quick and satisfying dessert or snack.

These guilt-free dessert recipes aim to provide
nutritious and delicious options for individuals
navigating breast cancer. As always, it's important
to consult with healthcare professionals regarding
specific dietary needs and preferences. Adjust the
recipes based on individual sensitivities and
preferences.

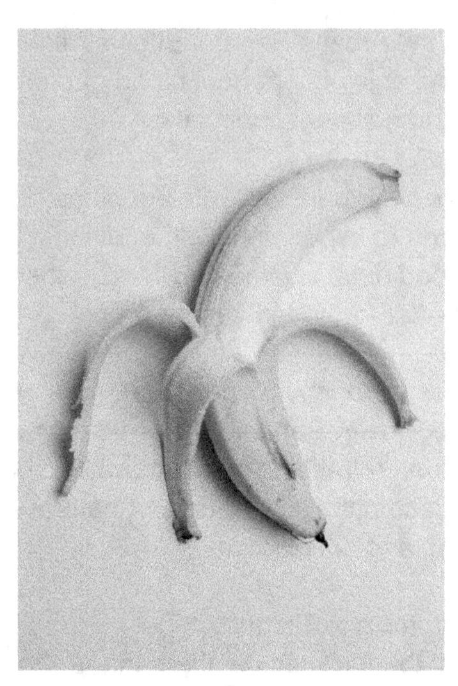

CHAPTER SEVEN

HYDRATION AND WELLNESS

Hydration is particularly important for individuals dealing with breast cancer, as it plays a crucial role in supporting overall wellness and can be essential during treatment. Here are considerations for hydration and wellness specifically tailored to individuals facing breast cancer:

Importance of Hydration during Breast Cancer:

1. **Treatment Side Effects:**
   - Certain cancer treatments, such as chemotherapy and radiation, may cause side effects like nausea, vomiting, and diarrhea, making it crucial to maintain hydration to manage these symptoms.

2. **Immune System Support:**
   - Staying well-hydrated supports the immune system, which is essential during cancer treatment to help the body cope with the effects of therapy.

3. **Energy Levels:**
   - Adequate hydration can help combat fatigue, a common side effect of cancer treatment, and improve overall energy levels.

4. **Nourishing the Body:**

- Proper hydration contributes to the nourishment of cells, supporting the body's ability to heal and recover.

5. **Digestive Health:**
   - Hydration is important for maintaining digestive health, particularly during times when the digestive system may be affected by cancer treatments.

Hydration Tips for Individuals with Breast Cancer:

1. **Regular Water Intake:**
   - Drink water regularly throughout the day. Sip small amounts consistently to maintain hydration.

2. **Hydrating Foods:**
   - Include hydrating foods in your diet, such as fruits with high water content (e.g., watermelon, oranges) and vegetables (e.g., cucumber, celery).

3. **Addressing Treatment Side Effects:**
   - If experiencing nausea or vomiting due to treatment, try sipping on clear fluids, such as water or ginger tea, and consult healthcare providers for guidance on managing symptoms.

4. **Electrolyte Balance:**
   - Consider beverages that help restore electrolyte balance, especially if experiencing dehydration from treatment side effects.

5. **Hydration and Physical Activity:**
   - Adjust hydration levels based on physical activity, taking into account any restrictions or recommendations from healthcare providers.

6. **Individualized Approach:**
   - Recognize that hydration needs are individual, and they may vary based on treatment, overall health, and individual circumstances.

7. **Hydration Journal:**
   - Keep a hydration journal to track daily fluid intake and identify patterns or adjustments that may be needed.

8. **Consult Healthcare Team:**
   - Always consult with the healthcare team for personalized advice on hydration, especially if facing treatment-related challenges.

Maintaining proper hydration is an important aspect of supporting overall wellness during the breast cancer journey. It can help manage treatment-related side effects, improve energy levels, and contribute to the body's resilience. Always seek guidance from healthcare professionals to address individual needs and challenges.

HEALING HERBAL TEAS AND INFUSION

While herbal teas and infusions are often enjoyed for their soothing qualities, it's crucial to note that they should not replace medical treatments prescribed by healthcare professionals. However, certain herbal teas may offer potential benefits and contribute to overall well-being. Here are some herbal teas and infusions that individuals with breast cancer might consider:

1. **Green Tea:**
   - **Potential Benefits:** Contains antioxidants, particularly catechins, which may have anti-cancer properties.
   - **Considerations:** Green tea contains caffeine, so moderation is advised, especially for those sensitive to caffeine.

2. **Turmeric Tea:**
   - **Potential Benefits:** Curcumin, the active compound in turmeric, has anti-inflammatory and antioxidant properties.
   - **Considerations:** Black pepper can enhance the absorption of curcumin, so consider combining turmeric with a pinch of black pepper.

3. **Ginger Tea:**
   - **Potential Benefits:** Known for its anti-nausea properties and may help alleviate digestive discomfort.

   - **Considerations:** Discuss with healthcare providers, especially if undergoing chemotherapy or taking blood-thinning medications.

4. **Chamomile Tea:**
   - **Potential Benefits:** Known for its calming properties and may help with sleep and relaxation.
   - **Considerations:** Some individuals may be allergic to chamomile, and it may interact with certain medications.

5. **Peppermint Tea:**
   - **Potential Benefits:** May help alleviate digestive issues and nausea.
   - **Considerations:** Peppermint can be refreshing, but some individuals may need to avoid it if they experience acid reflux.

6. **Holy Basil (Tulsi) Tea:**
   - **Potential Benefits:** Adaptogenic herb with potential stress-reducing properties.
   - **Considerations:** Consult with healthcare providers, especially if taking medications or managing blood sugar levels.

7. **Rosehip Tea:**
   - **Potential Benefits:** Rich in vitamin C and antioxidants, contributing to overall immune support.
   - **Considerations:** Avoid excessive intake, especially for those with kidney issues due to its oxalate content.

8. **Dandelion Root Tea:**
   - **Potential Benefits:** Traditionally used to support liver health, which may be relevant during cancer treatment.
   - **Considerations:** Discuss with healthcare providers, especially if experiencing liver issues or taking medications.

9. **Lemon Balm Tea:**
   - **Potential Benefits:** Known for its calming and anti-anxiety properties.
   - **Considerations:** May interact with certain medications, so discuss with healthcare providers.

10. **Hibiscus Tea:**
   - **Potential Benefits:** Rich in antioxidants, may contribute to heart health.
   - **Considerations:** Can lower blood pressure, so monitor levels if already low.

Tips for Herbal Teas:

- **Moderation is Key:** Consume herbal teas in moderation, and be mindful of individual reactions.

- **Consult Healthcare Providers:** Always consult healthcare providers, especially if undergoing cancer treatment or taking medications, as herbal teas may interact with medications or have contraindications.

- **Variety is Important:** Enjoy a variety of herbal teas rather than relying on a single type to benefit from a range of potential properties.

- **Listen to Your Body:** Pay attention to how your body responds to herbal teas and make adjustments accordingly.

Individual responses to herbs can vary, and what works for one person may not work for another. It's essential to approach herbal teas as complementary to conventional medical treatments and consult with healthcare providers for personalized advice based on individual health circumstances.

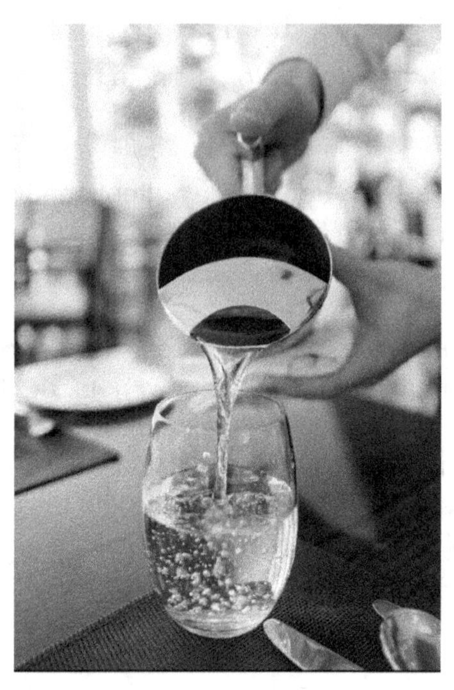

CHAPTER EIGHT

MEAL PLANNING AND PREP

Meal planning and preparation are excellent practices for maintaining a healthy and balanced diet, which is especially important during and after breast cancer treatment. The following advice can help you plan and prepare meals more effectively:

Meal Planning:

1. **Set Realistic Goals:**
   - Consider your energy levels and schedule when planning meals. Set objectives that are reasonable and in line with your present skills.

2. **Include a Variety of Foods:**
   - Aim for a diverse and colorful array of fruits, vegetables, whole grains, lean proteins, and healthy fats to ensure a well-rounded diet.

3. **Consider Dietary Preferences and Restrictions:**
   - Take into account personal preferences, dietary restrictions, and any guidance from healthcare providers when planning meals.

4. **Plan for Balanced Nutrients:**

- Ensure each meal includes a balance of protein, carbohydrates, healthy fats, vitamins, and minerals to support overall health.

5. **Portion Control:**
   - Take note of serving sizes to prevent overindulging. Consider using smaller plates to help with portion control.

6. **Prepare for Snacks:**
   - Include healthy snacks in your meal plan to keep energy levels steady throughout the day.

7. **Fluid Intake:**
   - Plan for adequate hydration by including water, herbal teas, and other hydrating beverages in your daily routine.

Meal Preparation:

1. **Batch Cooking:**
   - Prepare larger quantities of certain meals to have leftovers for future meals. This can save time and effort.

2. **Prep Ingredients in Advance:**
   - Wash, chop, and portion vegetables, fruits, and proteins in advance to streamline the cooking process during the week.

3. **Freezer-Friendly Meals:**

- Prepare meals that can be frozen for later use, providing convenience on days when cooking may be challenging.

4. **Simple and Nutrient-Dense Recipes:**
   - Focus on simple recipes with nutrient-dense ingredients to make meal preparation more manageable.

5. **Use Healthy Cooking Methods:**
   - Opt for healthier cooking methods such as baking, grilling, steaming, or sautéing, rather than deep-frying.

6. **Storage Organization:**
   - Invest in quality storage containers to keep prepared meals fresh. Label and date items for easy identification.

7. **Rotate Ingredients:**
   - Plan meals that share common ingredients to minimize waste and ensure you use perishables before they expire.

8. **Meal Prep Schedule:**
   - Establish a regular meal prep day each week to stay organized and ensure a steady supply of nutritious meals.

9. **Listen to Your Body:**
   - Observe how certain foods affect your body's reaction. Adjust your meal plan based on your

energy levels, appetite, and any dietary sensitivities.

Additional Considerations for Breast Cancer:

1. **Consult with Healthcare Providers:**
   - Consult with healthcare providers or a registered dietitian for personalized dietary recommendations based on your individual health status and any treatment-related considerations.

2. **Focus on Nutrient-Rich Foods:**
   - Emphasize foods that are nutrient-dense to support overall health and recovery.

3. **Adapt to Taste Changes:**
   - Be open to adapting recipes based on changes in taste preferences that may occur during and after treatment.

Remember, meal planning and preparation are tools to make your dietary choices more intentional and convenient. Adapt these tips to suit your preferences and lifestyle, and don't hesitate to seek guidance from healthcare professionals for personalized advice.

WEEKLY MEAL PLANS

Certainly! Here's a sample weekly meal plan with a variety of nutritious and balanced meals. Feel free to adjust portions and ingredients based on your preferences, dietary needs, and any guidance from healthcare providers.

Day 1:
Breakfast: Greek Yogurt Parfait with Mixed Berries and Granola

Lunch: Grilled chicken salad bowls

Dinner: Grilled lemon herb chicken

Snack: Sliced Apple with Almond Butter

Day 2:
Breakfast: Spinach and Feta Omelette with Whole Wheat Toast

Lunch: Lentil and Vegetable Soup with a Side of Whole Grain Crackers

Dinner: Quinoa and black bean burrito bowl

Snack: Greek Yogurt with Honey and a Handful of Mixed Nuts

Day 3:
Breakfast: Blueberry Almond Pancakes with a Dollop of Greek Yogurt

Lunch: Salmon and sweet potato

Dinner: Salmon and asparagus foil packets

Snack: protein packed energy bites

Day 4:
Breakfast: Chia Seed Pudding with Mango and a Sprinkle of Shredded Coconut

Lunch: Turkey and hummus whole wheat wrap

Dinner: Teriyaki Glazed salmon with sesame broccoli

Snack: Cottage Cheese and pineapple

Day 5:
Breakfast: Avocado and Egg Toast with Whole Grain Bread

Lunch: Mediterranean Chickpea Bowl with Mixed Greens and Lemon-Tahini Dressing

Dinner: Spinach and feta stuffed chicken breast

Snack: Trail Mix Power Bowl with Nuts and Dried Fruits

Day 6:
Breakfast: Peanut Butter Banana Toast with Chia Seeds

Lunch: Caprese wrap

Dinner: Salmon and Asparagus foil packets

Snack: avocado toast with poached eggs

Day 7:
Breakfast: Berry Power Smoothie with Spinach and Protein Powder

Lunch: Shrimp and avocado wrap

Dinner: chickpea and vegetable stir-fry

Snack: hummus and veggie sticks

Remember to stay hydrated throughout the day, incorporating water, herbal teas, or infused water with slices of citrus or cucumber. Adjust portion sizes based on your individual needs, and consider consulting with healthcare providers or a registered dietitian for personalized guidance.

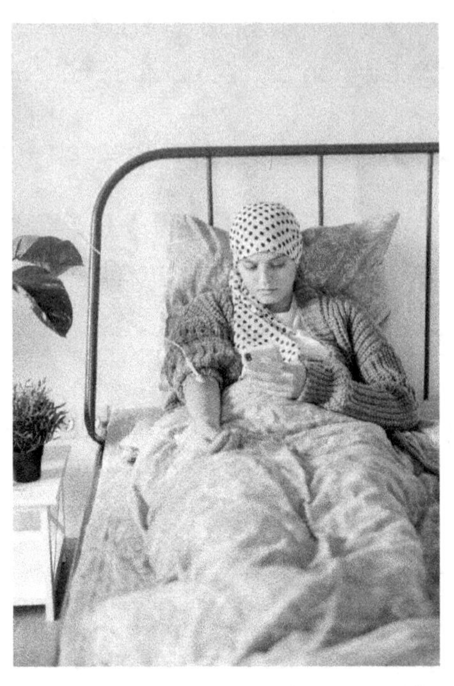

CHAPTER NINE

EMOTIONAL AND SOCIAL ASPECTS

Addressing the emotional and social aspects is crucial for overall well-being, especially during and after breast cancer treatment. Here are considerations for navigating these aspects:

Emotional Aspects:

1. **Seek Emotional Support:**
   - Share your feelings with loved ones, friends, or support groups. Having a supportive network can provide comfort and understanding.

2. **Professional Support:**
   - Consider talking to a mental health professional or counselor who specializes in supporting individuals dealing with cancer. They can provide coping strategies and a safe space to express emotions.

3. **Express Yourself Creatively:**
   - Engage in creative activities such as writing, drawing, or journaling to express your emotions and reflect on your journey.

4. **Mindfulness and Relaxation Techniques:**

- Practice mindfulness, meditation, or
deep-breathing exercises to help manage stress
and promote emotional well-being.

5. **Accept and Acknowledge Feelings:**
   - Experiencing a variety of emotions is natural.
Allow yourself to feel and acknowledge these
emotions without judgment.

6. **Set Realistic Expectations:**
   - Set realistic expectations for yourself,
recognizing that it's okay not to be okay at times.
Allow yourself the space to heal emotionally.

Social Aspects:

1. **Open Communication:**
   - Communicate openly with friends and family
about your needs, both emotionally and practically.
Tell them how you would like them to help.

2. **Join Support Groups:**
   - Connect with breast cancer support groups or
survivor networks. Sharing experiences with others
who understand can foster a sense of community
and validation.

3. **Educate Your Support System:**
   - Educate your support system about breast
cancer, treatment, and potential side effects. This
can enhance understanding and empathy.

4. **Social Outings:**
   - Take part in enjoyable social activities. Whether it's a casual outing with friends or a hobby you enjoy, maintaining social connections is vital.

5. **Boundary Setting:**
   - Set boundaries when needed. It's okay to communicate your comfort levels and prioritize self-care.

6. **Celebrate Milestones:**
   - Celebrate milestones, both big and small. Acknowledge achievements and positive moments in your journey.

7. **Stay Connected Digitally:**
   - Use digital platforms to stay connected with friends and family, especially if in-person interactions are limited.

8. **Educate Others:**
   - If comfortable, educate others about breast cancer, dispelling myths and promoting awareness. This can contribute to a supportive environment.

9. **Self-Advocacy:**
   - Advocate for your needs and preferences. Let others know how they can best support you emotionally and socially.

10. **Transitioning After Treatment:**

- Recognize that transitioning back to a "normal" life after treatment may come with its own set of challenges. Be patient with yourself and communicate your needs during this phase.

Remember, everyone's emotional and social journey is unique. Tailor these suggestions to your personal preferences and circumstances. If needed, professional counselors, support groups, or social workers can offer valuable guidance and resources.

COPING WITH CHANGES IN APPETITE

Coping with changes in appetite, whether it's an increase or decrease, is a common challenge during and after breast cancer treatment. Here are strategies to navigate these changes:

Decreased Appetite:

1. **Frequent, Smaller Meals:**
   - Try eating smaller, more frequent meals throughout the day in instead of three large ones. This can be less overwhelming and still provide necessary nutrients.

2. **Nutrient-Dense Foods:**
   - Focus on nutrient-dense foods that pack a lot of essential vitamins and minerals in smaller portions.

This ensures you get the most benefit from what you eat.

3. **Hydration:**
   - Stay well-hydrated. Sipping on water, herbal teas, or diluted fruit juices can be a good way to consume fluids without feeling overly full.

4. **High-Calorie Snacks:**
   - Include high-calorie snacks between meals, such as nuts, seeds, and dried fruits, to increase caloric intake without having to eat large quantities.

5. **Protein-Rich Foods:**
   - Prioritize protein-rich foods to support muscle strength and overall health. Options include lean meats, fish, eggs, dairy, legumes, and plant-based proteins.

Increased Appetite:

1. **Balanced Meals:**
   - Focus on balanced meals with a mix of proteins, healthy fats, and complex carbohydrates to promote satiety.

2. **Portion Control:**
   - Be mindful of portion sizes to avoid overeating. To give the impression that the plate is fuller, use smaller bowls and dishes.

3. **Choose Nutrient-Dense Snacks:**

- Opt for nutrient-dense snacks like fresh fruits, vegetables, yogurt, or whole-grain crackers to satisfy hunger without excessive calories.

4. **Mindful Eating:**
   - Practice mindful eating. Pay attention to hunger and fullness cues, and eat slowly to give your body time to register that it's satisfied.

5. **Hydration:**
   - Drink water before meals, as thirst can sometimes be mistaken for hunger. For general health, it is imperative to stay hydrated.

Coping Strategies for Both:

1. **Variety in Foods:**
   - Include a variety of foods to make meals more interesting and appealing. Try a variety of flavors, textures, and culinary styles.

2. **Adapt to Taste Changes:**
   - If taste changes are affecting your appetite, try different seasonings or spices to enhance flavors.

3. **Social Eating:**
   - Share meals with friends or family. Socializing during meals can create a positive environment and make eating more enjoyable.

4. **Multivitamin Supplements:**

- If it's challenging to get all the necessary nutrients from food, talk to your healthcare team about the possibility of taking a multivitamin supplement.

5. **Listen to Your Body:**
   - Observe how various foods affect your body's reaction. If certain foods are well-tolerated and enjoyable, incorporate them into your diet.

6. **Consult with a Dietitian:**
   - Seek guidance from a registered dietitian specializing in oncology nutrition. They can provide personalized advice based on your individual needs and preferences.

Remember, changes in appetite are normal, and it's essential to be patient with yourself. If these changes persist or significantly impact your well-being, discuss them with your healthcare team, as they can provide additional guidance and support.

SHARING MEALS WITH LOVED ONES

Sharing meals with loved ones is a wonderful way to foster connections and create meaningful experiences. Here are some tips for making these shared meals enjoyable, especially during and after breast cancer treatment:

Planning and Preparation:

1. **Collaborative Meal Planning:**
   - Involve loved ones in meal planning. This not only shares the responsibility but also allows everyone to contribute their preferences and ideas.

2. **Consider Dietary Preferences and Restrictions:**
   - Take into account any dietary preferences or restrictions, including those related to breast cancer treatment. Plan meals that cater to everyone's needs.

3. **Simple and Flexible Recipes:**
   - Opt for simple recipes with flexible ingredients. This allows for customization based on individual preferences and dietary requirements.

4. **Delegate Tasks:**
   - Delegate tasks during meal preparation. Everyone can contribute by chopping vegetables, setting the table, or preparing a specific part of the meal.

Creating a Comfortable Environment:

1. **Set a Welcoming Table:**
   - Create a warm and inviting atmosphere by setting a nicely decorated table with fresh flowers

or candles. This can make the meal feel more special.

2. **Choose Comfortable Seating:**
   - Ensure seating arrangements are comfortable and conducive to conversation. Consider cushions or throws for added coziness.

3. **Background Music:**
   - Put on some calming background music to improve the atmosphere. Choose music that everyone can enjoy and that complements the mood.

Emphasizing Connection:

1. **Engaging Conversations:**
   - Encourage open and engaging conversations during the meal. Share stories, memories, and thoughts to create a sense of connection.

2. **Device-Free Time:**
   - Consider having device-free time during the meal. This allows everyone to be fully present and engaged in the shared experience.

3. **Expressing Gratitude:**
   - Take a moment to express gratitude for the shared time and the effort put into the meal. This can foster a positive and appreciative atmosphere.

Flexibility and Understanding:

1. **Be Flexible with Timing:**
   - Be flexible with meal timing to accommodate everyone's schedules. It's about the shared experience, not the rigid adherence to a specific mealtime.

2. **Understand Preferences:**
   - Understand and respect individual food preferences. If someone has specific dietary needs or restrictions, accommodate those with alternative options.

Making it Special:

1. **Celebrate Milestones:**
   - Use shared meals as an opportunity to celebrate milestones, whether big or small. It could be a personal achievement, a special occasion, or simply the joy of being together.

2. **Try New Recipes Together:**
   - Experiment with trying new recipes together. This can be a fun and collaborative activity that adds an element of adventure to the shared meal experience.

Remember, the essence of sharing meals with loved ones is the connection and shared joy. Tailor these tips to fit your unique circumstances, and enjoy the moments of togetherness around the table.

CONCLUSION

In conclusion, the journey through breast cancer involves various dimensions, including physical, emotional, and social aspects. Navigating these challenges requires a holistic approach that addresses both the medical and personal dimensions of the experience. As highlighted in this breast cancer cookbook, the importance of nutrition, emotional well-being, and social support cannot be overstated.

Understanding the impact of breast cancer on appetite, meal planning, and emotional and social aspects is crucial. Coping with changes in appetite, whether an increase or decrease, involves mindful choices, adaptability, and seeking support when needed. Additionally, the emotional and social aspects of the journey are integral to overall well-being, emphasizing the significance of communication, understanding, and the support of loved ones.

Sharing meals with loved ones becomes a poignant and supportive aspect of this journey. The act of coming together around the table fosters connection, celebration, and a shared sense of strength. By embracing flexibility, understanding, and the joy of creating positive experiences, meals become not just a source of nourishment but a symbol of resilience and togetherness.

In this cookbook, we've aimed to provide a diverse range of recipes that cater to nutritional needs, varying appetites, and the desire for flavorful, enjoyable meals. From breakfast boosters to satisfying dinners and guilt-free desserts, the recipes are crafted with care, keeping in mind the importance of nourishing the body and the spirit.

As you embark on this journey, remember that every individual's experience is unique. Adapt these recipes and suggestions to suit your preferences and circumstances. Consult with healthcare professionals for personalized guidance, and above all, approach each meal with a sense of self-care and compassion.

May this cookbook serve as a companion in your journey, offering nourishment, support, and the reminder that you are not alone. Your strength, resilience, and the love of those around you are integral parts of the recipe for well-being. Wishing you healing, joy, and moments of shared warmth around the table.